BRITISH MEDICAL BULLETIN

Type 2 diabetes: the thrifty phenotype

Scientific Editor: *David J P Barker*

http://www.bmb.oupjournals.org

Acknowledgements

The planning committee for this issue of the *British Medical Bulletin* was chaired by David Barker and also included Nick Hales, Abigail Fowden and David Phillips.

The British Council and Oxford University Press are most grateful to them for their help and advice and for the valuable work of the Scientific Editor in completing this issue.

Preface

Like other living creatures, human beings are 'plastic' in early life: their growth and development are moulded by the environment. Although the growth of the fetus is driven by the generative programme contained in its genome, it is limited by the supply of nutrients from the mother. There are many reasons why it may be advantageous, in evolutionary terms, for the body's structure and function to remain plastic in early life and this is a general phenomenon of early development.

The human baby responds and adapts to the nutrients it receives by altering its production of hormones and the sensitivity of its tissues to them, by changing its metabolism, and by redistributing its cardiac output to protect key organs, especially the brain. Slowing of growth is adaptive because it reduces the requirements for substrate. Unlike physiological adaptations in adulthood, those made during development tend to lead to life-long changes in the structure and function of the body – a phenomenon sometimes referred to as programming. It is as though the baby receives from its mother a forecast of the nutritional environment it will encounter after birth and changes its physiology and metabolism accordingly.

The plasticity of human development has been known for a long while. Only recently, however, has evidence appeared suggesting that the origins of important chronic diseases of adult life, including coronary heart disease, stroke and type 2 diabetes may lie in fetal responses to the intra-uterine environment. The 'fetal origins' hypothesis proposes that these disorders originate through adaptations which the fetus makes when it is malnourished. A feature of the early findings, which came mainly from epidemiological studies, was the strength of the associations between small body size at birth and later disease. Important biological effects must underlie such associations, and it soon became evident that these effects could be replicated experimentally in animals, usually by reducing the mother's food intake around the time of conception and during pregnancy.

This book focuses on the links between early growth and type 2 diabetes, more specifically the insulin resistance syndrome, in which insulin resistance and impaired glucose tolerance are combined with hypertension and dyslipidaemia. Ten years ago, a study in Hertfordshire, England, showed for the first time that people who had had low birthweight were more insulin resistant and had higher rates of type 2 diabetes in later life. This association has been confirmed in studies in Europe, the US and other countries. We now need to understand the processes that underlie it, and this is the subject of this book.

The first chapter by Hales & Barker describes the 'thrifty phenotype' hypothesis. It proposes that type 2 diabetes originates in poor nutrition in fetal life and infancy, which lead to insulin resistance and accompanying changes in glucose and lipid metabolism. The baby thereby becomes adapted to poor nutrition and is 'thrifty'. For so long as it continues to be poorly nourished during childhood and adult life, these adaptations are beneficial. With increased food intake, decreased energy expenditure and the development of obesity, however, the adaptations are no longer beneficial. Increased insulin resistance, combined with a reduced capacity to secrete insulin because of impaired pancreatic β-cell development, lead to impaired glucose tolerance, and ultimately to the insulin resistance syndrome and type 2 diabetes.

A key issue is to what extent does the association between low birthweight and type 2 diabetes reflect poor nutrition or other environmental influences in early life, and to what extent does it reflect genetic influences. Lindsay & Bennett argue for the importance of genes and re-state the 'thrifty genotype' hypothesis. 40 years ago, Neel proposed that predisposition to type 2 diabetes might arise through genetic variations that were favourable in times when malnutrition was widespread but became unfavourable as nutrition improved. Caroline Fall addresses the rising epidemics of type 2 diabetes that are now occurring in the non-industrialised world. Are the poorer peoples of the world doomed by their genetic inheritance? Or can the adverse effects of increasing energy intakes be offset by improved fetal and infant nutrition? Whatever the answer there is no doubt that obesity is a driving force in these epidemics and we need to know more about the gene–environment interactions which underlie it. These are discussed in the next chapter by Andrew Prentice.

In discussion of nutrition in early life, the distinction between fetal and maternal nutrition is sometimes not made, and maternal nutrition is simply equated with the mother's diet in pregnancy. In the next chapter I describes how a mother's ability to nourish her baby is established during her own fetal life and by her nutritional experiences in childhood and adolescence, which determine her body size, composition and metabolism. While the supply of nutrients to the fetus is known to be the major influence that regulates its growth, Frayling & Hattersley argue for the importance of genetic influences in determining the links between size at birth and later disease.

A strength of the fetal origins hypothesis is that it is supported by experimental findings. Experiments show that even minor modifications to the diet of female animals before and during pregnancy may be followed by life-long changes in the offspring in ways that can be related to human disease – for example altered glucose-insulin metabolism and elevated blood pressure. This is the subject of the next five chapters. Bertram & Hanson describe animal models that have been used to study programming. Fowden & Hill review programming of the endocrine pancreas. Metabolic programming is reviewed by Susan Ozanne, while Christopher Byrne describes the programming of two hormonal axes that modulate insulin action, the hypothalamic-pituitary-adrenal axis and the growth hormone-insulin-like growth factor axis. The long-term consequences of the abnormal intra-uterine environment associated with maternal diabetes are described by Van Assche, Holemans & Aerts.

Finally, Eriksson, Lindström & Tuomilehto return us to public health. Research into the thrifty phenotype hypothesis has two goals. One of them is to determine whether the rising epidemics of type 2 diabetes can be lessened by improving the body composition and nutrition of girls and young women and by protecting the growth of young children. The other goal is the earlier detection and better treatment of the disease. To realise both goals, clinicians, basic scientists and epidemiologists must join forces. My thanks go to the contributors to this book, who have done just that in order to write it. Thanks also to my colleagues, Shirley Simmonds and Pam Freeman, who helped with the editing, and to Gill Haddock who produced the book.

D J P Barker

The thrifty phenotype hypothesis

C Nicholas Hales* and **David J P Barker†**

*Department of Clinical Biochemistry, University of Cambridge, Addenbrooke's Hospital, Cambridge, UK and †MRC Environmental Epidemiology Unit, Southampton General Hospital, Southampton, UK

The thrifty phenotype hypothesis proposes that the epidemiological associations between poor fetal and infant growth and the subsequent development of type 2 diabetes and the metabolic syndrome result from the effects of poor nutrition in early life, which produces permanent changes in glucose-insulin metabolism. These changes include reduced capacity for insulin secretion and insulin resistance which, combined with effects of obesity, ageing and physical inactivity, are the most important factors in determining type 2 diabetes. Since the hypothesis was proposed, many studies world-wide have confirmed the initial epidemiological evidence, although the strength of the relationships has varied from one study to another. The relationship with insulin resistance is clear at all ages studied. Less clear is the relationship with insulin secretion. The relative contribution of genes and environment to these relationships remains a matter of debate. The contributions of maternal hyperglycaemia and the trajectory of postnatal growth need to be clarified.

*Correspondence to:
Prof. C N Hales,
Department of Clinical
Biochemistry, University
of Cambridge,
Addenbrooke's Hospital,
Hills Road, Cambridge
CB2 2QR, UK*

The thrifty phenotype hypothesis[1] was put forward 10 years ago in an attempt to explain the associations between poor fetal and infant growth and increased risk of developing impaired glucose tolerance[2] and the metabolic syndrome[3] in adult life. Figures 1 and 2 show the original findings of these associations among men in Hertfordshire[2,3]. In the intervening years, many data have emerged showing the reproducibility of these epidemiological findings in different populations and ethnic groups. The validity of the findings is now generally accepted. A key matter for debate is to what extent the underlying mechanisms explaining the links are genetic or environmental. It is clear that genetic causes of poor insulin secretion can be associated with poor fetal growth, though they are rare (*see* Frayling & Hattersley, this issue). This is not in principle surprising, since insulin is a major fetal growth hormone. There is some indication that other genetic polymorphisms may be linked to birth weight and subsequent changes in glucose metabolism[4], but these effects are considerably less strong than the effect of birth weight itself[5]. It is facile to state that the pathogenesis of type 2 diabetes resides in a mixture of genetic and environmental factors, since this is true of every

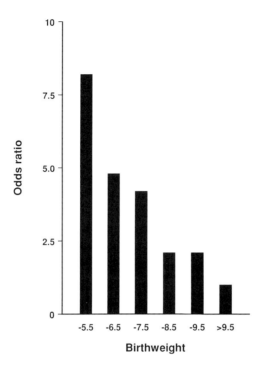

Fig. 1 Odds ratio for impaired glucose tolerance or type 2 diabetes according to birth weight among 370 men aged 64 years born in Hertfordshire (adjusted for adult body mass index).

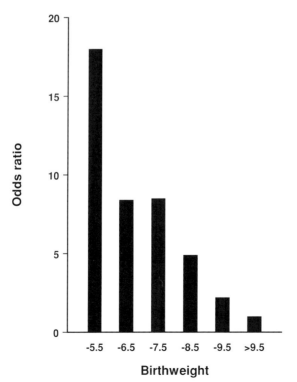

Fig. 2 Odds ratio for the metabolic syndrome according to birth weight among 407 men born in Hertfordshire (adjusted for adult body mass index).

human characteristic. Genetic factors are known to be involved in diseases such as tuberculosis and malaria, but the only credible approach to their prevention and treatment is to attack their major environmental cause – infection. It is, therefore, important to establish whether environmental factors acting in early life play a major role in the pathogenesis of type 2 diabetes.

The thrifty phenotype hypothesis proposes that environmental factors are the dominant cause of type 2 diabetes. In this chapter, we shall summarise the hypothesis as originally proposed; review the human and animal data which have emerged subsequently; consider, in the light of this how the hypothesis should be refined; and finally present what we believe are the key issues to be tackled by future research.

The thrifty phenotype hypothesis

Figure 3 shows the original diagrammatic representation of the thrifty phenotype hypothesis. The central element is that poor fetal and infant nutrition are the insult that drives the process. World-wide, the most important cause of malnutrition in early life is maternal malnutrition (*see* Barker, this issue). However, other influences, maternal and placental, may also be involved. A contribution of malnutrition in infancy was included because of our finding that the link between low weight at 1 year and the subsequent risk of glucose intolerance among men could not be explained simply by the strong association between weight at 1 year and birth weight. In considering the downstream effects of poor fetal nutrition, we proposed that poor development of pancreatic β-cell mass and function (including islet of Langerhans vasculature and possibly innervation) were key elements linking poor early nutrition to later type 2 diabetes. We also suggested that fetal malnutrition led to insulin resistance. Fetal nutrition thereby set in train mechanisms of fetal nutritional thrift, which had a differential impact on the growth of different organs, with selective protection of brain growth. Altered growth permanently changes the structure and function of the body.

A poor functional capacity for insulin secretion would not be detrimental to individuals who continued to be poorly nourished and remained thin and, therefore, insulin-sensitive. Glucose intolerance would be triggered by a positive calorie balance as a result of increased food intake and decreased energy expenditure leading to obesity. The combination of malnutrition during fetal life and infancy followed by overnutrition in childhood and adult life characterises populations undergoing the transition from chronic malnutrition to adequate nutrition (*see* Fall, this issue). The thrifty phenotype hypothesis postulated a key role for protein supply because of the extensive

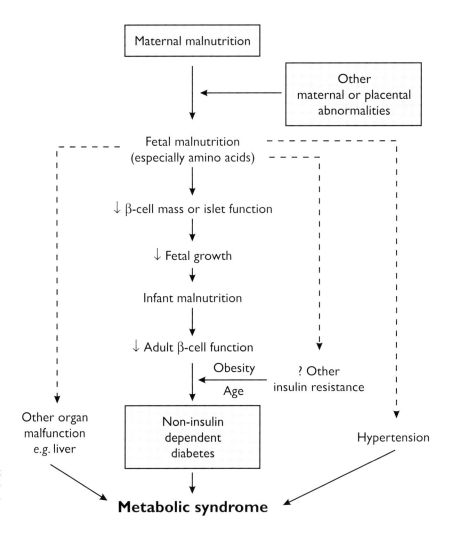

Fig. 3 The original diagrammatic representation of the thrifty phenotype hypothesis.

literature on this aspect of nutrition, but other nutritional deficits were not excluded. Indeed the variety of combinations of metabolic changes seen in patients with the metabolic syndrome might be accounted for by a variety of combinations and timings of nutritional deficiencies in fetal life and infancy. The hypothesis also proposed that the emergence of pathological changes following undernutrition in early life was critically dependent upon the superimposition of other factors, notably obesity, ageing and physical inactivity.

We suggested that those interested in candidate genes for type 2 diabetes should widen their horizons and consider genes involved in fetal growth and development. Since then mutations in transcription factors relevant to β-cell development have been shown to be a cause of maturity onset diabetes of the young, albeit a rare cause. Gene defects which reduce fetal insulin production and polymorphisms of the insulin gene itself, are associated with type 2 diabetes and exemplify the crucial role of early development in determining the disease.

Recent studies

Body size at birth and the metabolic syndrome

Since the original descriptions of the relationships between birth weight or thinness at birth, indicated by a low ponderal index (birth weight/length^3) and the later development of type 2 diabetes and the metabolic syndrome,

Table 1 Populations in which relationships between birth weight, shortness or thinness at birth and altered glucose and insulin metabolism or the metabolic syndrome have been described

	Age (years)
Indian children	4[6]
Pima Indians (USA)	5–29[7]
Black South African children	7[8]
Jamaican school children	6–10[9]
Salisbury children (UK)	7[10]
Prepubertal children (New Zealand)	8.5[11]
British children	10–11[12]
Italian children	8–14[13]
Southampton men (UK)	18–25[14]
French adults	21[15]
Australian men	21[16]
Danish men and women	18–32[17]
British pregnant women	27[18]
Pima Indians (USA)	20–38[19]
Mexican Americans and non-Hispanic whites	32[20]
Indian men and women	39–60[21]
Health professional men (USA)	40–75[22]
Oxford men and women (UK)	43[23]
Chinese men and women	45[24]
Danish men and women	48[25]
Preston men and women (UK)	46–54[26]
Preston men and women	47–55[27]
Swedish men	40–60[28]
Swedish men	50–76[29]
Dutch men and women	50[30]
Postmenopausal women (USA)	50–84[31]
Sheffield men and women (UK)	52[32]
Danish twins	55–74[33]
Hertfordshire men (UK)	55–74[2]
Nurses' health study (women USA)	59[34]
British women	65[35]
Swedish men	70[36]

these findings have been replicated in a variety of populations around the world (Table 1). We are not aware of any study which contradicts them. In considering the impact of poor fetal growth on later type 2 diabetes, a number of factors have to be taken into account. Birth weight or thinness at birth are but poor surrogates for the estimate of the success of a pregnancy. Weight alone does not reveal the relative contributions of fat mass and lean body mass. It was clear from the early studies of men in Hertfordshire that in this population there was a continuous relationship between birth weight and glucose tolerance. There was no threshold. Thus it is incorrect to argue that since in the Western world low birth weight is rare the impact of poor fetal growth on the risk of diabetes must, therefore, be small. Whatever the factors may be which low birth weight is signalling as being important in determining the risk of type 2 diabetes, they operate across the range of birth weights. Whilst they may operate most intensely in low birth weight babies, they also operate in the much greater number of babies who fall within what we consider to be the 'normal' birth weight range. It is, therefore, important that we try to define the phenotypes of growth-retarded babies at risk of later type 2 diabetes as precisely as possible. The hope is that animal experiments will reveal in detail, at the level of gene and protein expression, just what aspects of metabolism are programmed in association with reduced early growth.

Glucose tolerance itself is determined by both insulin secretion and insulin sensitivity. In epidemiological studies, the relationship of poor early growth to subsequent insulin resistance is much clearer and stronger than it is to poor insulin secretion. The latter has been observed in young men but not in older populations. In the elderly, the effects of life-long insulin resistance may have caused adaptive changes to insulin secretion, which obscure its relationship with early growth restriction. The relative roles of insulin secretion and sensitivity appear to differ between individuals. There are indications that men tend to be more insulin-resistant than women and the converse in relation to insulin secretion. This could represent sexual dimorphism in response to a similar insult. In experimental animals, there are large differences in the impact of poor maternal nutrition on the relative growth of different organs in males and females.

Childhood growth and the metabolic syndrome

A question arising from the association between type 2 diabetes and small body size at birth is whether, or to what extent, the increased risk of the disease associated with reduced prenatal growth is modified by particular patterns of growth throughout childhood. Suggestive evidence that childhood growth may be important comes from a study showing that obesity in childhood has a greater effect on the development of the

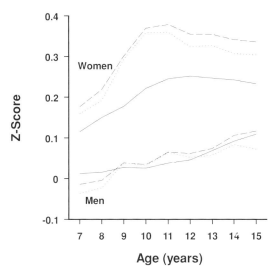

Fig. 4 Height, weight and body mass index (BMI) during childhood of 286 men and 185 women who later developed type 2 diabetes. The solid line indicates height; dashed line indicates weight; dotted line indicates body mass index.

metabolic syndrome than does obesity that occurs in adulthood[37]. The detailed information on body size at birth and during childhood that is available in a cohort of 7086 men and women born in Helsinki, Finland, allows the issue to be addressed directly[38]. Figure 4 shows the childhood growth of the 471 men and women who developed type 2 diabetes. Height, weight and body mass index (weight/height^2) are expressed as standard deviation or so-called Z-scores. These represent the differences, expressed in standard deviations, from the mean value for the whole cohort, which is set at zero. Children maintaining a steady position as large or small in relation to other children would follow a horizontal path on the figure. Children who later developed type 2 diabetes, however, having been short or thin at birth continued to have low rates of growth in infancy, as was found in Hertfordshire[2], but from 7 years onwards had accelerated growth in weight and height. By the age of 15 years, boys and girls who later developed type 2 diabetes were above the average for the cohort in weight and body mass index. Data from a second Helsinki Cohort, which includes growth measurements between birth and 7 years, show that the accelerated weight gain began at 2 years of age (manuscript in preparation). Accelerated weight gain had a greater effect on increased risk of type 2 diabetes among men and women who weighed 3000 g or less at birth. It occurred among children born to heavier mothers with higher body mass indices, suggesting that it resulted from high energy intakes in childhood. In families where the mother was well-nourished it seems likely that there would have been more food available to the children.

The processes through which accelerated childhood weight gain increases the risk of type 2 diabetes are not known. It does not seem to be through worsening of insulin resistance. Examination of 500 men and women from an older cohort, born in Helsinki during 1924–1933[39], showed that the development of insulin resistance was associated with thinness at birth and continued thinness in childhood, followed by the development of overweight in adult life. One possible explanation for the adverse effect of accelerated weight gain is that fetal growth restriction leads to reduced cell numbers in the endocrine pancreas and subsequent accelerated growth in childhood leads to excessive metabolic demand on this limited cell mass.

Famine and the metabolic syndrome

The role of accelerated child growth in the genesis of type 2 diabetes may explain the differing results of the effects of wartime famine in Holland[30] and Leningrad[40]. The famine in western Holland began abruptly in November 1944 and ended abruptly with the liberation of Holland in May 1945. Men and women exposed to the famine while they were *in utero* had higher plasma glucose concentrations 2 h after a standard glucose load. They also had higher fasting pro-insulin and 2 h plasma insulin concentrations, which suggests that their poor glucose tolerance was partly determined by insulin resistance. The 'Dutch famine' is unique in that it was a brief period of intense deprivation in a well-nourished population whose level of nutrition was promptly restored after the famine. Children exposed to famine *in utero* were, therefore, well-nourished in childhood and could have had accelerated weight gain.

In contrast, the siege of Leningrad occurred over a prolonged period, 1941–1944, in a previously malnourished population who remained badly nourished after the siege was lifted. Children probably did not have accelerated weight gain. This (together with the small size of the Leningrad study) offers one explanation of why the associations between famine exposure and altered glucose-insulin metabolism, although in the expected direction, were small and not statistically significant.

Consistent with other studies, the people in the Dutch study who had low birth weight had raised 2 h plasma glucose concentrations, but the effects of famine were largely independent of this. One explanation is that the initial adaptation of the fetus to undernutrition is to alter its metabolism, including its glucose-insulin metabolism, and continue to grow. Only if these adaptations fail does it reduce its rate of growth. Whatever the explanation, the findings from the Dutch famine are important because they provide direct evidence that undernutrition *in utero* leads to impaired glucose tolerance and type 2 diabetes, and they show that the mother's dietary intake during pregnancy can programme metabolism without altering size at birth. Because of its brief duration, the Dutch famine provides information about the effects of fetal undernutrition at different stages of gestation. The findings require confirmation in further studies, but it seems that famine exposure in early gestation led to disturbance of lipid metabolism while in mid and late gestation it led to disturbance of glucose-insulin metabolism.

Genes versus the environment

Whilst there is now little dispute that indices of poor early growth are linked to increased risk of impaired glucose tolerance and the metabolic syndrome, the extent to which genes or the early environment underlie the relationship remains controversial. We have argued elsewhere that the evidence linking a genetic cause to the aetiology of type 2 diabetes is poorly founded[41]. Studies of identical twins (which spuriously initiated the current preoccupation with the genetic causes of type 2 diabetes) have shown that poor fetal growth operates to increase the risk of the condition independently of the genetic constitution[42]. On the other hand, recent studies of paternal effects on birth weight and subsequent diabetes have been interpreted as evidence of genetic causation[43].

Time trends

Experience on the Pacific Island of Nauru gives an insight into how improving nutrition may be associated with a rise in type 2 diabetes followed by a fall[44]. The island population was chronically malnourished until the end of the Second World War. The flourishing phosphate mines built up after the war drastically changed the economic and nutritional welfare of the population. The immediate consequence of this was a great increase in obesity and the emergence of an 'epidemic' of type 2 diabetes. However, subsequent studies of individuals born after the war in better nutritional circumstances (but for whom unfortunately we do not have birth weights or infant weights) have shown a substantial reduction in glucose intolerance[44]. This population is particularly informative because over the years of study the amount of obesity, although great, has not increased. In contrast, in the Western world obesity is increasing and, until this trend ceases or is reversed, the benefits of improved fetal and infant growth may not be evident in declining rates of type 2 diabetes.

Animal models

Investigations in animals to examine the mechanisms and results of altered fetal and early postnatal nutrition are described elsewhere in this issue (experiments specifically designed to test and elaborate on the thrifty phenotype hypothesis in rats are described by Ozanne). Poor fetal growth may result from a variety of causes. It is not clear whether the long-term phenotypic consequences of the different causes of reduced fetal growth are the same, varied or totally discrepant. Intuitively it seems likely, but is by no means clearly established, that the consequences of fetal growth restriction will vary according to the stage of pregnancy at which they operate, and findings in the Dutch famine studies encourage this view. Equally it seems likely that different nutritional influences will lead to different phenotypic results. Studies of the latter question are still at an early stage. At the present time, however, what is most apparent is the relative consistency of results irrespective of the type of insult provided. Perhaps it would not be altogether surprising if the fetus had a limited range of responses. While the use of reduced maternal protein intake as an experimental model in animals may not reflect the commonest problem facing human populations, it may evoke common fetal responses to undernutrition. This may explain why this specific and limited nutritional deficiency induces a phenotype with such remarkable parallels to the human metabolic syndrome and type 2 diabetes. In continuing animal studies, we need more specific molecular markers of changes in gene expression to examine this question. Whole body markers of change such as glucose tolerance and blood pressure have an inherent wide variability demanding the use of large numbers of animals to define end points.

In parallel with the human studies already described, studies of the effects of postnatal growth in animals have revealed relevant and potentially interesting changes. The longevity of male rats is linked to their pattern of early growth: female rats show the same pattern, but much smaller differences. Male rats which had been growth restricted during fetal life, having been produced by a dam fed a reduced protein diet, but who had accelerated growth postnatally, by being cross fostered to normally fed lactating dams and weaned onto a normal diet fed *ad libitum*, died young (13.1 months of age compared with controls 15.1 months). The converse pattern was observed in male pups born to a normally fed mother but who were then cross-fostered onto low protein fed dams (mean age at death 17.0 months). They suffered considerable growth restriction whilst suckling, but surprisingly when weaned onto a normal diet fed *ad libitum* they did not 'catch up' in growth, remaining permanently growth restricted[45]. We were able to show that this growth restriction was accompanied by a reduced food intake. One explanation of this is that nutrition during suckling 'sets' appetite. If the nutrition of rat litters is manipulated, by changing litter sizes, this permanently changes food intake even after weaning. Good nutrition, produced by culling litters to small numbers, leads to animals with an increased appetite. Poor nutrition, produced by expanding the litter with additional pups from other newly delivered animals, leads to animals with a decreased appetite.

The hypothesis updated

Whilst we are not aware of data from epidemiological studies or animal research which contradict any of the key features of the thrifty phenotype hypothesis, as originally proposed, it is clear that with increased insight into the biological processes, the content and precision of the hypothesis can be improved. Our current understanding of the links between maternal malnutrition and fetal malnutrition is described elsewhere (*see* Barker, this issue), which also describes the inter-generational effects of poor maternal nutrition.

Consequences of fetal malnutrition

It has become apparent that the consequences of fetal malnutrition on organ growth differ in males and females. Animal studies have indicated that as well as changes in organ size there may be substantial changes in organ structure. Offspring of low protein fed dams have livers with larger but fewer lobules. Even within these lobules, the gradient of cell types observed going from the periportal to the perivenous zones seems to have been altered. Such changes must have profound implications for the varied functions of the liver, which include the production of acute phase proteins, now well recognised as being changed in type 2 diabetes.

It has become increasingly apparent that the response to fetal malnutrition entrains not only (presumably advantageous) selective preservation of key organs but also metabolic adaptations of advantage for postnatal survival. Thus the thrifty phenotype is not only thrifty with respect to antenatal life, but also in relation to the use of poor nutritional resources postnatally. The poorly nourished mother essentially gives the fetus a forecast of the nutritional environment into which it will be born. Processes are set in motion which lead to a postnatal metabolism adapted to survival under conditions of poor nutrition. The adaptations only become detrimental when the postnatal environment differs from the mother's forecast, with an over abundance of nutrients and consequent obesity. Similar observations have been made in relation to cold exposure. Offspring of sheep exposed to cold during pregnancy are, on delivery, better adapted to respond to cold conditions after birth.

The altered metabolic features of the offspring of rat dams fed a low protein diet are reviewed elsewhere in this issue (*see* Van Assche *et al*). These include increased hepatic gluconeogenesis, enhanced release of fatty acids from intra-abdominal adipose tissue, resistance to ketosis and increased expression of insulin receptors with enhanced uptake of glucose by adipose tissue. These are all features which could be expected to be advantageous to an animal exposed to poor nutrition in postnatal life.

An updated version of the diagrammatic representation of the thrifty phenotype hypothesis is shown in Figure 5. Also included in the diagram are more speculative suggestions that changes in the structure and function of blood vessels may play a key role in changing organ growth and function, and that maternal hyperglycaemia may contribute to the type and consequences of fetal malnutrition.

Future research

Continuing observational epidemiological studies are required to address two questions. First, what are the influences which, acting

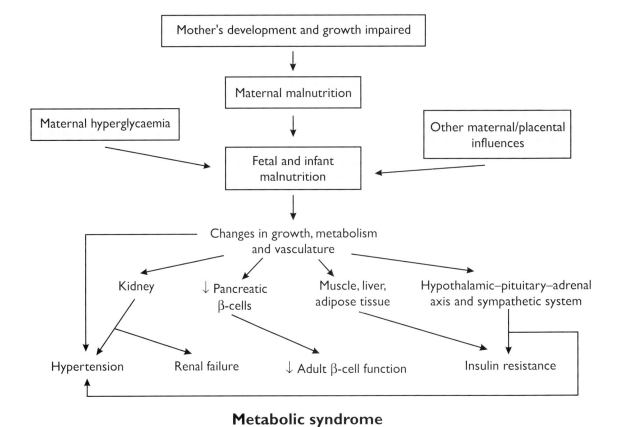

Fig. 5 An updated diagram of the thrifty phenotype hypothesis incorporating recent findings and concepts. Also included are new speculative features: maternal hyperglycaemia as predisposing factor and key roles of the vascular, hypothalamic-pituitary-adrenal axis and sympathetic systems.

through the mother or directly on the infant after birth, permanently change the body's structure and metabolism in ways which lead to type 2 diabetes? Second, how do these changes in structure and metabolism alter the body's responses to adverse influences in later life? The importance of the first question is self-evident; the second is proving a fruitful area of research. We now know that the effects of rapid weight gain in childhood, and obesity in adult life, on increased risk of type 2 diabetes is greater among men and women who had low birth weight. It is likely that many such interactions between body size in early life and influences acting in later life will be discovered.

As is argued in the preface, sufficient is now known to plan intervention studies and new public health policies. These will be refined as new information comes forward from clinical and animal studies.

More research needs to be done in animals to document the consequences of nutritional growth restriction. Few organs and systems have been studied in detail. It is also apparent that the effect of age is important, but few studies have been carried out on ageing animals – largely because of the facilities and time required. Provision needs to be made for such long-term studies. The range of animals studied remains narrow – rodents, guinea pigs and sheep. Little or no work has been carried out in primates and there is an obvious need for this. Experimental models of fetal growth restriction used have been limited. There is a need for the use of common end-points and their application to a range of relevant causes of growth restriction. It is far from clear how much phenotypic variability results from different types and timings of fetal and postnatal growth restriction. More needs to be known about the beneficial or detrimental effects of accelerated postnatal growth and how its impact varies with the stage in postnatal life at which it occurs.

Finally, and most crucially in relation to advancing human studies, we need molecular markers at the protein and RNA level which specifically define malnutrition at different stages of fetal life and infancy. These must first be uncovered in animal studies because of the limited nature of what can be done in humans. However, once these have been defined and tested in animals there will be great potential for them to refine and expedite human studies and, hopefully, reduce the number of subjects required. It should be possible to define end points in early postnatal life so that the success of intervention studies can be established more rapidly.

Conclusions

In the interval since the proposal of the thrifty phenotype hypothesis, the epidemiological data which led to its formulation have received substantial and widespread international confirmation. There is a continuing debate as to the relative importance of genetic *versus* environmental factors in determining fetal growth and subsequent adult susceptibility to type 2 diabetes and the metabolic syndrome. Studies of identical twins show conclusively that the fetal environment is important. There is a major need for molecular markers of metabolic programming in fetal life. When these are available, it will be simpler to monitor at an early stage the success of intervention studies. We believe that the thrifty phenotype hypothesis continues to provide a useful conceptual framework within which to design and interpret human and animal studies in this field.

References

1   Hales CN, Barker DJP. Type 2 (non-insulin-dependent) diabetes mellitus: the thrifty phenotype hypothesis. *Diabetologia* 1992; **35**: 595–601
2   Hales CN, Barker DJP, Clark PMS *et al*. Fetal and infant growth and impaired glucose tolerance at age 64. *BMJ* 1991; **303**: 1019–22
3   Barker DJP, Hales CN, Fall CHD, Osmond C, Phipps K, Clark PMS. Type 2 (non-insulin-dependent) diabetes mellitus, hypertension and hyperlipidaemia (syndrome X): relation to reduced fetal growth. *Diabetologia* 1993; **36**: 62–7
4   Dunger DB, Ong KK, Huxtable SJ *et al*. Association of the INS VNTR with size at birth. ALSPAC Study Team Avon longitundinal study of pregnancy and childhood. *Nat Genet* 1998; **19**: 98–100
5   Ong KK, Phillips DI, Fall C *et al*. The insulin gene VNTR, type 2 diabetes and birth weight. *Nat Genet* 1999; **21**: 262–3
6   Yajnik CS, Fall CHD, Vaidya U *et al*. Fetal growth and glucose and insulin metabolism in four-year-old Indian children. *Diabet Med* 1995; **12**: 330–6
7   Dabelea D, Pettitt DJ, Hanson RL, Imperatore G, Bennett PH, Knowler WC. Birth weight, type 2 diabetes, and insulin resistance in Pima Indian children and young adults. *Diabet Care* 1999; **22**: 944–50
8   Crowther NJ, Cameron N, Trusler J, Gray IP. Association between poor glucose tolerance and rapid post natal weight gain in seven-year-old children. *Diabetologia* 1998; **41**: 1163–7
9   Forrester TE, Wilks RJ, Bennett FI *et al*. Fetal growth and cardiovascular risk factors in Jamaican schoolchildren. *BMJ* 1996; **312**: 156–60
10 Law CM, Gordon GS, Shiell AW, Barker DJP, Hales CN. Thinness at birth and glucose tolerance in seven-year-old children. *Diabet Med* 1995; **12**: 24–9
11 Hofman PL, Cutfield WS, Robinson EM *et al*. Insulin resistance in short children with intrauterine growth retardation. *J Clin Endocrinol Metab* 1997; **82**: 402–6
12 Whincup PH, Cook DG, Adshead F *et al*. Childhood size is more strongly related than size at birth to glucose and insulin levels in 10–11-year-old children. *Diabetologia* 1997; **40**: 319–26
13 Chiarelli F, di Ricco L, Mohn A, Martino M, Verrotti A. Insulin resistance in short children with intrauterine growth retardation. *Acta Paediatr Suppl* 1999; **428**: 62–5
14 Robinson S, Walton RJ, Clark PM, Barker DJP, Hales CN, Osmond C. The relation of fetal growth to plasma glucose in young men. *Diabetologia* 1992; **35**: 444–6
15 Leger J, Levy-Marchal C, Bloch J *et al*. Reduced final height and indications for insulin resistance in 20 year olds born small for gestational age: regional cohort study. *BMJ* 1997; **315**: 341–7
16 Flanagan DE, Moore VM, Godsland IF *et al*. Fetal growth and the physiological control of glucose tolerance in adults: a minimal model analysis. *Am J Physiol Endocrinol Metab* 2000; **278**: E700–6

17 Clausen JO, Borch-Johnsen K, Pedersen O. Relation between birth weight and the insulin sensitivity index in a population sample of 331 young, healthy Caucasians. *Am J Epidemiol* 1997; **146**: 23–31

18 Olah KS. Low maternal birth weight – an association with impaired glucose tolerance in pregnancy. *J Obstet Gynaecol* 1996; **16**: 5–8

19 McCance DR, Pettitt DJ, Hanson RL, Jacobsson LTH, Knowle WC, Bennett PH. Birth weight and non-insulin dependent diabetes: 'thrifty genotype', 'thrifty phenotype', or 'surviving small baby genotype'. *BMJ* 1994; **308**: 942–5

20 Valdez R, Athens MA, Thompson GH, Bradshaw BS, Stern MP. Birth weight and adult health outcomes in a biethnic population in the USA. *Diabetologia* 1994; **37**: 624–31

21 Fall CHD, Stein CE, Kumaran K *et al*. Size at birth, maternal weight, and type 2 diabetes in South India. *Diabet Med* 1998; **15**: 220–7

22 Curhan GC, Willett WC, Rimm EB, Spiegelman D, Ascherio AL, Stampfer MJ. Birth weight and adult hypertension, diabetes mellitus, and obesity in US men. *Circulation* 1996; **94**: 3246–50

23 Cook JTE, Levy JC, Page RCL, Shaw JAG, Hattersley ATG, Turner RC. Association of low birth weight with β cell function in the adult first degree relatives of non-insulin dependent diabetic subjects. *BMJ* 1993; **306**: 302–6

24 Mi J, Law C, Zhang K-L, Osmond C, Stein C, Barker D. Effects of infant birth weight and maternal body mass index in pregnancy on components of the insulin resistance syndrome in China. *Ann Intern Med* 2000; **132**: 253–60

25 Vestbo E, Damsgaard EM, Frøland A, Mogensen CE. Birth weight and cardiovascular risk factors in an epidemiological study. *Diabetologia* 1996; **39**: 1598–602

26 Phipps K, Barker DJP, Hales CN, Fall CHD, Osmond C, Clark PMS. Fetal growth and impaired glucose tolerance in men and women. *Diabetologia* 1993; **36**: 225–8

27 Phillips DIW, Barker DJP, Hales CN, Hirst S, Osmond C. Thinness at birth and insulin resistance in adult life. *Diabetologia* 1994; **37**: 150–4

28 Carlsson S, Persson PG, Alvarsson M *et al*. Low birth weight, family history of diabetes, and glucose intolerance in Swedish middle-aged men. *Diabetes Care* 1999; **22**: 1043–7

29 Lithell HO, McKeigue PM, Berglund L, Mohsen R, Lithell U-B, Leon DA. Relation of size at birth to non-insulin dependent diabetes and insulin concentrations in men aged 50–60 years. *BMJ* 1996; **312**: 406–10

30 Ravelli ACJ, van der Meulen JHP, Michels RPJ *et al*. Glucose tolerance in adults after prenatal exposure to famine. *Lancet* 1998; **351**: 173–7

31 Yarbrough DE, Barrett-Connor E, Kritz-Silverstein D, Wingard DL. Birth weight, adult weight, and girth as predictors of the metabolic syndrome in postmenopausal women: the Rancho Bernardo Study. *Diabetes Care* 1998; **21**: 1652–8

32 Martyn CN, Hales CN, Barker DJP, Jespersen S. Fetal growth and hyperinsulinaemia in adult life. *Diabet Med* 1998; **15**: 688–94

33 Poulsen P, Kyvik KO, Vaag A, Beck-Nielsen H. Heritability of type 2 (non-insulin-dependent) diabetes mellitus and abnormal glucose tolerance – a population-based twin study. *Diabetologia* 1999; **42**: 139–45

34 Rich-Edwards JW, Colditz GA, Stampfer MJ *et al*. Birth weight and the risk for type 2 diabetes mellitus in adult women. *Ann Intern Med* 1999; **130**: 278–84

35 Fall CHD, Osmond C, Barker DJP *et al*. Fetal and infant growth and cardiovascular risk factors in women. *BMJ* 1995; **310**: 428–32

36 McKeigue PM, Lithell HO, Leon DA. Glucose tolerance and resistance to insulin-stimulated glucose uptake in men aged 70 years in relation to size at birth. *Diabetologia* 1998; **41**: 1133–8

37 Vanhala M, Vanhala P, Kumpusalo E, Halonen P, Takala J. Relation between obesity from childhood to adulthood and the metabolic syndrome: population based study. *BMJ* 1998; **317**: 319

38 Forsen T, Eriksson J, Tuomilehto J, Reunanen A, Osmond C, Barker DJP. The fetal and childhood growth of persons who develop type 2 diabetes. *Ann Intern Med* 2000; **133**: 176–82

*40 Eriksson J, Forsen T, Jaddoe VWV, Osmond C, Barker DJP. The effects of childhood growth and maternal body size on insulin resistance in elderly men and women. *Diabelologica 2002*; In press

41 Stanner SA, Bulmer K, Andres C *et al.* Does malnutrition *in utero* determine diabetes and coronary heart disease in adulthood? Results from the Leningrad siege study, a cross sectional study. *BMJ* 1997; **315**: 1342–8

42 Hales CN, Desai M, Ozanne SE. The thrifty phenotype hypothesis: how does it look after 5 years? *Diabet Med* 1997; **14**: 189–95

43 Poulsen P, Vaag AA, Kyvik KO, Moller Jensen D, Beck-Nielsen H. Low birth weight is associated with NIDDM in discordant monozygotic and dizygotic twin pairs. *Diabetologia* 1997; **40**: 439–46

44 Lindsay RS, Dabelea D, Roumain J, Hanson RL, Bennett PH, Knowler WC. Type 2 diabetes and low birth weight: the role of paternal inheritance in the association of low birth weight and diabetes. *Diabetes* 2000; **49**: 445–9

45 Dowse GK, Zimmet PZ, Finch CF, Collins VR. Decline in incidence of epidemic glucose intolerance in Nauruans: implications for the 'thrifty genotype'. *Am J Epidemiol* 1991; **133**: 1093–104

46 Hales CN, Desai M, Ozanne SE, Crowther NJ. Fishing in the stream of diabetes: from measuring insulin to the control of fetal organogenesis. *Biochem Soc Trans* 1996; **24**: 341–50

Type 2 diabetes, the thrifty phenotype – an overview

Robert S Lindsay and **Peter H Bennett**

National Institute of Diabetes and Digestive and Kidney Diseases, National Institutes of Health, Phoenix, Arizona, USA

Searching for the causes of type 2 diabetes

Diabetes mellitus is a group of metabolic disorders characterized by chronic hyperglycaemia[1]. Within this group, type 2 diabetes describes the form of the disease usually with onset in adult life, and associated with insulin resistance and relative insulin deficiency, as opposed to the absolute deficiency found in type 1 diabetes[1]. Type 2 diabetes is of great importance to public health due to the burden of morbidity and mortality associated with this common disease[2].

Type 2 diabetes is a complex disorder likely to have multiple genetic and environmental causes. Enormous efforts are being made to discover the genetic determinants of the disease. Recently, important additions have been made to our knowledge of the physiology of glucose and energy homeostasis at the molecular level – major advances have been made in our understanding of the mechanisms of insulin action, insulin secretion and control of appetite and energy balance[3,4]. In addition, the genetic causes of a number of relatively rare causes of diabetes and obesity – one of the major known risk factors for development of type 2 diabetes – have been discovered, such as the multiple forms of maturity onset diabetes of the young (MODY)[5] and mutations in leptin[6] and the leptin receptor[7], as rare genetic causes of human obesity. It seems likely that these advances, along with efforts to positionally clone candidate genes for type 2 diabetes in a number of populations, will lead in the near future to discovery of the major sources of genetic variation which predispose individuals to develop type 2 diabetes.

At the same time, current evidence confirms the continuing, and at the population level increasing, importance of environmental factors in the development of type 2 diabetes and obesity. The prevalences of these two conditions are rising in populations world-wide[2,8]. These increases in prevalence are clearly not caused by changes in the genetic make up of these populations, but indicate the importance of the environment in the development of type 2 diabetes and obesity, and that exposure to adverse environments is increasing. Some of the environmental factors are well known. Availability of calorie rich diets and secular decreases in

Correspondence to:
Dr Peter H Bennett,
National Institute of
Diabetes and Digestive
and Kidney Diseases,
1550 East Indian School
Road, Phoenix,
AZ 85014, USA

habitual physical activity have been noted in a number of populations and undoubtedly contribute to the increasing prevalence of obesity and, in turn, type 2 diabetes[8]. Ultimately, the cause of type 2 diabetes is likely to reflect a mix of genetic and environmental causes and, importantly, interactions between genes and environment. In this context, environmental causes of type 2 diabetes, including low levels of physical activity and availability of calorie rich diets, are undoubtedly of major importance. The subject of this issue of this book, however, concerns the evidence for other environmental risk factors, in particular whether environmental factors in early life contribute to later development of type 2 diabetes.

The thrifty phenotype

The thrifty phenotype hypothesis, introduced by Hales and Barker in 1992[9], proposed the concept that environmental factors acting in early life, in particular undernutrition, might influence later risk of type 2 diabetes. The hypothesis arose, in large part, from the pioneering work of the MRC Environmental Epidemiology Unit in Southampton which, under the directorship of David Barker, explored the geographical and socio-economic distributions of chronic diseases[10]. In particular, they were interested in the temporal relationships of socio-economic conditions and vascular disease: historically, cardiovascular disease was more prevalent in more affluent socio-economic groups, but over time this association appeared to become inverted such that cardiovascular disease became more prevalent in poorer parts of society in countries like the UK. This was linked with the paradox that while on a world-wide basis cardiovascular disease might be considered a disease of 'affluence', being concentrated in more prosperous nations, within some of those societies rates of cardiovascular disease were generally highest in the least affluent parts of society[10]. This led to the investigation of relationships of early life experiences, measured by factors such as infant mortality and birth weight, to later cardiovascular disease[10].

An association of lower birth weight to later disease was first observed in relation to cardiovascular disease, and subsequently extended to cardiovascular risk factors. Relationships of low birth weight and type 2 diabetes were developed by Barker in collaboration with Hales[9], and termed the 'thrifty phenotype hypothesis'. Hales and Barker described the novel association of low birth weight with later development of type 2 diabetes in a cohort of men studied in Hertfordshire, England[11]. The original observations have now been replicated in several populations[12] and have been extended to examine important antecedents of type 2 diabetes including markers of insulin secretion[13] and insulin resistance[14].

Both the low birth weight and thrifty phenotype hypotheses were born into what might be considered a hostile environment, consequently they generated enormous controversy. Because of this, and their implications in several fields of medicine, the hypotheses will already be familiar to practitioners in endocrinology, cardiology and respiratory disease, but they also have broader implications important to other fields. Research stimulated by the thrifty phenotype hypothesis has led to an increased understanding of the plasticity of early human development, and highlighted how this plasticity might contribute to later human disease. The number of fields of medicine and basic biology influenced by these hypotheses is attested to by the range of topics included in this issue.

In this introduction, we will not recapitulate the evidence for and against the different parts of the thrifty phenotype hypothesis, as these topics are covered in detail in later chapters, but rather highlight the contribution we feel it has made to our understanding of the pathophysiology of diabetes and in stimulating further research.

Thrifty genotypes and thrifty phenotypes

While the theme of this issue is the thrifty phenotype, it is appropriate to first consider an older hypothesis – 'the thrifty genotype' – in contra-distinction to which the name of the 'thrifty phenotype' is derived. While overall, the two hypotheses are very different, they share important features. Both address the basic mechanisms which underlie the aetiology of such a common disease as type 2 diabetes. Both have been important in stimulating further research.

In 1962, Neel introduced the thrifty genotype hypothesis, addressing the aetiology of diabetes (the distinctions between type 1 and type 2 diabetes had not been defined at that time) and obesity from the perspective of evolutionary biology[15]. Neel proposed that predisposition to diabetes might arise because of genetic variations which were advantageous in certain environmental situations but were later rendered disadvantageous – and disease causing – in different environments. More specifically, that human variations which were favourable in populations facing challenges of episodic undernutrition might be disadvantageous when food supplies became abundant: in Neel's words[15] 'a thrifty genotype rendered detrimental by progress'. In particular, Neel proposed that the increased fat storage would be accomplished by alteration of the threshold and amount of insulin release in response to meals ('the fast insulin trigger') and that this predisposed to diabetes and obesity.

While much of the physiological basis provided in the original paper has been superseded[16], the general hypothesis has proven attractive in providing potential explanations for subsequent observations concerning the epidemiology of type 2 diabetes. Firstly, as type 2 diabetes is such a common condition, it seems plausible that genetic variation predisposing to diabetes might have been associated with selective advantage at some point over the course of human evolution. Neel's hypothesis suggests one potential mechanism for this. Secondly, it provides a possible explanation for why the propensity to diabetes varies greatly among populations. The prevalence of type 2 diabetes is profoundly different in different ethnic groups. The highest known prevalence of type 2 diabetes occurs in the Pima Indian population of Arizona, among whom over 60% of adults develop the disease[17]. Other American Indian groups as well as Polynesian and Micronesian populations also have very high prevalence of type 2 diabetes, followed by migrant Asian Indians[2]. Undoubtedly some of these differences relate to non-genetic factors, particularly with regard to contemporary environmental influences on physical activity and nutritional intake. It is also likely that differences in underlying genetic predisposition to type 2 diabetes exist between ethnic groups. Again, Neel's hypothesis provides a potential explanation for this: differences in genetic predisposition to diabetes being the result of different forces of selection due to nutritional circumstance in the various populations.

The thrifty phenotype hypothesis proposes a very different aetiological model for type 2 diabetes. In this model, undernutrition acts not as a selection pressure acting over many generations to alter the genetic make up of the population, but rather as an early environmental influence acting in an individual to increase risk of type 2 diabetes[9]. In Neel's hypothesis, entire populations have an increased predisposition to type 2 diabetes – because of genetic selection, they are better adapted to different nutritional circumstances than those they experience today. In the thrifty phenotype hypothesis, maladaptive responses occur as a result of environmentally induced alteration of physiology in the early life of the individual. Both hypotheses offer explanations of why the frequency of diabetes and obesity may differ in different populations and why predisposition to diabetes is common, albeit by very different mechanisms.

Early environmental Influence before and after the thrifty phenotype

The basic concept advanced by the thrifty phenotype hypothesis is that human disease may arise due to early environmental effects whose influence to cause disease is only expressed much later in life. Thus, the influences of the environmental exposure are not confined to the time frame in which they are experienced but may continue to act through the life of the organism and long after an adverse exposure has ended. As a further refinement of this hypothesis, it is proposed that certain key developmental windows exist during which exposures 'set' physiological systems and thus lead to long-term consequences. This concept has been termed[18] environmental 'programming'.

When the thrifty phenotype hypothesis was proposed, this concept was not new to the field of metabolic disease in humans. The importance of the early environment had already been invoked as an explanation of increased propensity to diabetes in offspring of diabetic mothers – a very different early nutritional model to that proposed in the thrifty phenotype hypothesis. As early as 1960, White made fundamental observations regarding the high prevalence of abnormal glucose tolerance in offspring of diabetic mothers[19]. Around the same time, Pedersen developed the hypothesis that early **overexposure** to glucose *in utero* resulted in organomegaly and excessive growth that might then predispose to subsequent diabetes[20]. Frienkel then extended this hypothesis to propose that overexposure to a range of intermediary metabolites, most importantly glucose and amino acids, might act in the long-term to alter metabolism and lead to human disease[21], a concept he termed fuel mediated teratogenesis. Pettitt and colleagues then showed that both obesity[22] and type 2 diabetes[23] were more prevalent in the offspring of mothers who had had diabetes during pregnancy- suggesting that predisposition to these conditions had arisen as a consequence of the intra-uterine environment.

Similarly, in the field of obesity it had already been proposed that influences in early life might be important in later predisposition to obesity. In 1972, Brook proposed that obesity might be influenced by events *in utero*[24], following the concept of the time that adipocyte differentiation occurred primarily in the intra-uterine period. Stein and Susser explored the influence of early undernutrition, due to exposure to war time famine, on later predisposition to obesity, finding that exposure to famine early in intra-uterine life was associated with an increase in later obesity[25].

A variety of observations and hypotheses regarding long-term influences of hormonal exposure on endocrine axes had also been established in experimental animals. The best known of these is the example of plasticity in the hypothalamic–pituitary–gonadal axis. Since the 1960s, it had been recognized that there is a 'window' in the first 10 days of post-natal life in which exposure of a new-born female rat to a single pulse of testosterone leads to reduced fertility in adult life[26]. This arises because androgen exposure or non-exposure at this stage of development permanently alters hypothalamic responses to a male or female pattern respectively[26,27], a phenomenon the authors called 'imprinting', borrowing the term from behavioural psychology[28].

The thrifty phenotype hypothesis has also been important in stimulating later, different hypotheses addressing how the environment in early life might act to influence later disease. The presence or absence of breast feeding in early life has been proposed to influence later development and predisposition to disease. Pettitt *et al* observed that breast-feeding in the first 2 months of life was associated with a lower risk of development of type 2 diabetes in the Pima population[29]. Such a protective effect of breast-feeding has also been observed for childhood obesity[30].

Challenges to the thrifty phenotype

In part, the evidence for the thrifty phenotype rests upon the observation of associations of later human disease and lower birth weight. Initially, this basic observation was widely challenged, but has now been replicated in several separate studies and populations. More recently others, most notably Hattersley, have explored whether that association might arise not because of environmental insults *in utero*, but because of a genetic connection between lower birth weight and later diabetes[31], as discussed elsewhere in this issue. Maturity onset diabetes of the young (MODY) was originally described as a syndrome of early onset non-insulin dependent diabetes with a clinical features more typical of type 2 than type 1 diabetes and with an autosomal dominant pattern of inheritance[32]. It is now known that MODY is caused by a range of genetic mutations[5]. Hattersley *et al* demonstrated that one of the causes of MODY – mutation of the glucokinase gene – when present in the fetus is also associated with lower birth weight as well as later diabetes[33]. While the frequency of this mutation is too low to explain the associations seen in the populations described by Barker and Hales, it does demonstrate the potential for genetic mechanisms to underpin associations of birth weight and later disease. Insulin is a major promoter of growth *in utero*[31]. Consequently, genes which affect either insulin secretion or insulin resistance might well influence both fetal growth and subsequently development of diabetes[31]. Indeed, disruption of a variety of genes involved in insulin secretion or signalling, such as IRS-2, are known in animal models to result in alteration of fetal growth[34]. Does variation in such genes result in alteration of birth weight in human populations? At present, the evidence is limited, although in a single study common variants of several candidates genes did not appear to influence birth weight[35].

Our own work has also examined whether genetic influences might underpin some of the associations of birth weight and diabetes in the American Indian populations. The Pima population of Arizona have an extremely high prevalence of obesity and type 2 diabetes – an increase that is believed to reflect both current environmental influences, such as

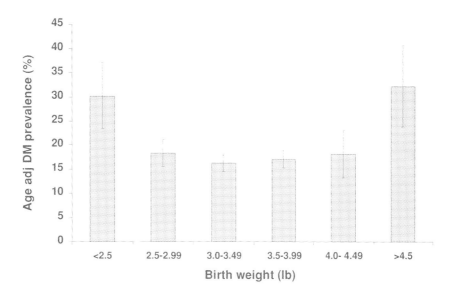

Fig. 1 The relation of birth weight and later prevalence of type 2 diabetes in the Pima population. Prevalence of type 2 diabetes is adjusted for age using the direct method using the age distribution of 1179 subjects, and presented as mean and 68% confidence intervals. Redrawn from McCance et al[36].

reduced levels of exercise and inappropriately high caloric intake, as well as genetic predisposition to both type 2 diabetes and obesity. In the Pima, we have demonstrated that both low and high birth weight are associated with an increased later risk of type 2 diabetes (Fig. 1)[36]. High birth weight principally reflects influences of maternal diabetes in pregnancy both to increase birth weight and to increase likelihood of type 2 diabetes in later life[37]. As an alternative to both the thrifty genotype and thrifty phenotype hypotheses, we have suggested that the association of low birth weight with type 2 diabetes in the Pima population might reflect selective survival of low birth weight infants, with genetically determined metabolic characteristics that were also related to the later development of diabetes[36]. Such an advantage *in utero* and infancy could represent a powerful selective force over the course of human evolution.

More recently, we have examined relationships of parental diabetes to low birth weight. If the association between low birth weight and later diabetes is due to genetic effects, then the parents of low birth weight offspring should themselves be at a greater risk of diabetes[38]. Conversely, the absence of such effects would be more consistent with the notion that early environmental influences were a cause of diabetes in these lower birth weight offspring. In the Pima, lower birth weight is indeed associated with

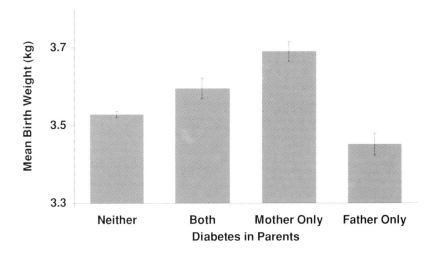

Fig. 2 Mean birth weight of children divided by last known diabetes status of their parent. Groups: Neither, neither parent ever diagnosed with diabetes; Both, both parents diagnosed with diabetes; Mother Only and Father Only, mother or father diabetic. respectively, second parent non-diabetic. Values are expressed as mean ± SEM. General linear model consistent with a significant effect of parental diabetes diagnosis on birth weight (*P* <0.001) and independent effects of both maternal (*post hoc* Student Newman Keuls, *P* <0.0001) and paternal (Student Newman Keuls, *P* < 0.001) diabetes status. Redrawn from Lindsay *et al*[38].

parental diabetes, but in fact solely with diabetes in fathers (Fig. 2). Furthermore, the ability of low birth weight to predict later diabetes in offspring appears to depend on the presence of diabetes in fathers[38]. These observations appear to strengthen the case for a genetic link between low birth weight and type 2 diabetes. The particular association with paternal diabetes has also led us to consider whether genomic imprinting – differential expression of genes depending on parent of origin – might be a determining factor in the low-birth weight diabetes relationship[38]. Imprinting is known to act in syndromic causes of obesity and diabetes such as Prader-Willi syndrome and transient neonatal diabetes mellitus (TNDM: OMIM 601410). Intriguingly, the majority of currently recognised imprinted genes appear to influence pathways involving fetal growth or placental development[39,40]. If low birth weight is associated with type 2 diabetes secondary to genetic influences, might this arise through actions of imprinted genes on both fetal growth and glucose homeostasis? Others have made similar proposals. Recently, type 2 diabetes has been associated with a genetic polymorphism on chromosome 11p found close to the insulin gene (INS VNTR III), but only if the associated allele was transmitted from the father[41]. The authors concluded that an imprinted gene in this region might be acting to increase the risk of type 2 diabetes[41].

The role of genes and environment in determining associations of low birth weight with later disease is by no means settled. The strictly genetic interpretation is challenged by twin studies of Poulsen *et al* who have demonstrated that in identical twins the smaller twin is more likely to develop type 2 diabetes[42]. Given that identical twins share all of their genes, the authors interpret this as evidence that an environmental effect acting on the smaller twin is increasing risk of metabolic disease – lending support to the environmental hypothesis of Hales and Barker. On the other hand, a recent report of a considerably larger series of monozygotic twins (together with a contemporary series of dizygotic twins) failed to find any relationship between birth weight and either blood pressure or glucose intolerance among the twin pairs[43]. This report casts doubt on the hypothesis that environmental effects on intra-uterine growth *per se* are important determinants of low birth weight-blood pressure and low birth weight-glucose intolerance relationships.

A second challenge to the thrifty phenotype hypothesis comes from those who accept the importance of early environmental influences on both birth weight and later disease, but question whether undernutrition is the specific critical environmental determinant. The role of nutrition in altering pancreatic insulin secretion and insulin resistance had been addressed by a large number of studies in animal models – some of which are reviewed in this issue. A number of human populations who have been subject to periods of undernutrition because of deprivation during World War II have also been examined to assess whether maternal undernutrition during pregnancy resulted in long-term consequences for the children. Children born during famine in Holland (survivors of 'the Dutch Hunger Winter') were found to have significantly higher 2-h plasma glucose concentrations[44]. By contrast, children whose mothers survived the siege of Leningrad appeared to have no long-term effect on blood glucose, although the authors comment on the difficulty of ascertaining the extent of exposure to famine in this group, especially when pregnant women may have had preferential access to food[44]. (Further discussion of these two war-time famines is given by Prentice in this issue.) While the Dutch study would support the hypothesis that undernutrition during pregnancy can lead to metabolic consequences, the second raises doubts as to whether such effects may only be exerted in the most extreme circumstances, making undernutrition unlikely to be instrumental in the aetiology of most cases of type 2 diabetes. Other authors have sought to explain the findings of low birth weight in terms of other early environmental insults, including the actions of glucocorticoids *in utero* to increase predisposition to type 2 diabetes[45].

Why is the thrifty phenotype hypothesis important? Future challenges

We do not know yet how great a role early nutrition plays in the generation of later diabetes. One cannot doubt, however, the enormous importance of the thrifty phenotype hypothesis in stimulating research examining the aetiology of this common disease.

The high prevalence of type 2 diabetes seen in many populations lends additional importance to both the thrifty phenotype and thrifty genotype. On a clinical level, any hypothesis attempting to understand the aetiology of such a common disease is important if new understanding emanates which helps to prevent or treat the disease in the future. On a more fundamental level, it is hard to believe that the mechanisms underlying such a common disease will not also reflect upon normal physiology. If fetal programming is a key mechanism in the generation of diabetes, it is likely that such a mechanism will play a part in programming normal metabolism – with implications for other aspects of physiology. The thrifty phenotype has also stimulated researchers to re-address concepts of the plasticity of human responses, hormonal and physiological, in the face of environmental insults and the way that such insults may exert permanent effects on the organisms. It serves to remind us that despite the recent triumphs of genetics and molecular biology, an understanding of environmental influences and how genes and the environment interact is likely to be critical to our understanding of many common, chronic human diseases. Finally, and of greatest challenge to the medical and public health community, if early environment influences later disease, it obliges all health professionals involved in early human development to re-appraise their goals. Perhaps in the future we will have to place more emphasis on the long-term, and possibly unexpected, effects of interventions taken in early life. Early environmental influences on later disease may carry implications for all clinicians, but may be most important for those who develop health policy addressing the health and nutrition of mothers and children.

References

1   World Health Organization. Diabetes mellitus. Report of a WHO Study Group. *WHO Technical Report Series* 1985; No. 727
2   Amos AF. The rising global burden of diabetes and its complications: estimates and projections to the year 2010. *Diabet Med* 1997; **14 (Suppl 5)**: S1–85
3   Shepherd PR. Glucose transporters and insulin action – implications for insulin resistance and diabetes mellitus. *N Engl J Med* 1999; **341**: 248–57
4   Friedman JM. Leptin and the regulation of body weight in mammals. *Nature* 1998; **395**: 763–70
5   Hattersley AT. Maturity-onset diabetes of the young: clinical heterogeneity explained by

genetic heterogeneity. *Diabet Med* 1998; **15**: 15–24

6   Montague CT, Farooqi IS, Whitehead JP *et al*. Congenital leptin deficiency is associated with severe early-onset obesity in humans. *Nature* 1997; **387**: 903–8

7   Clement K, Vaisse C, Lahlou N *et al*. A mutation in the human leptin receptor gene causes obesity and pituitary dysfunction. *Nature* 1998; **392**: 398–401

8   World Health Organization. Obesity: preventing and managing the global epidemic. Reprt of a WHO Consultation, *WHO Technical Report Series* 2000; No. 894

9   Hales CN, Barker DJ. Type 2 (non-insulin-dependent) diabetes mellitus: the thrifty phenotype hypothesis. *Diabetologia* 1992; **35**: 595–601

10 Barker DJP. Review: rise and fall of Western diseases. In: Barker DJP (ed). *Fetal and Infant Origins of Adult Disease*. London: BMJ Publishing, 1992

11 Hales CN, Barker DJ, Clark PM *et al*. Fetal and infant growth and impaired glucose tolerance at age 64. *BMJ* 1991; **303**: 1019–22

12 Hales CN, Desai M, Ozanne SE. The thrifty phenotype hypothesis: how does it look after 5 years? *Diabet Med* 1997; **14**: 189–95

13 Cook JT, Levy JC, Page RC, Shaw JA, Hattersley AT, Turner RC. Association of low birth weight with beta cell function in the adult first degree relatives of non-insulin dependent diabetic subjects. *BMJ* 1993; **306**: 302–6

14 Phillips DI, Barker DJ, Hales CN, Hirst S, Osmond C. Thinness at birth and insulin resistance in adult life. *Diabetologia* 1994; **37**: 150–4

15 Neel JV. Diabetes mellitus: a thrifty genotype rendered detrimental by 'progress'. *Am J Hum Genet* 1962; **14**: 353–62

16 Neel JV. The 'thrifty genotype' in 1998. *Nutr Rev* 1999; **57**: S2–9

17 Knowler WC, Pettitt DJ, Saad MF, Bennett PH. Diabetes mellitus in the Pima Indians: incidence, risk factors and pathogenesis. *Diabetes Metab Rev* 1990; **6**: 1–27

18 Lucas A. Programming by early nutrition in man. In: Bock G, Whelan J. (eds) *The Childhood Environment and Adult Disease*. Chichester: Wiley, 1991; 38–55

19 White PW. Childhood diabetes: its course and influence in the second and third generations. *Diabetes* 1960; **9**: 345–55

20 Pedersen J. Weight and length at birth in infants of diabetic mothers. *Acta Endocrinol* 1954; **16**: 330–42

21 Freinkel N. Banting Lecture 1980. Of pregnancy and progeny. *Diabetes* 1980; **29**: 1023–35

22 Pettitt DJ, Baird HR, Aleck KA, Bennett PH, Knowler WC. Excessive obesity in offspring of Pima Indian women with diabetes during pregnancy. *N Engl J Med* 1983; **308**: 242–5

23 Pettitt DJ, Aleck KA, Baird HR, Carraher MJ, Bennett PH, Knowler WC. Congenital susceptibility to NIDDM. Role of intrauterine environment. *Diabetes* 1988; **37**: 622–8

24 Brook CG. Evidence for a sensitive period in adipose-cell replication in man. *Lancet* 1972; **2**: 624–7

25 Ravelli GP, Stein ZA, Susser MW. Obesity in young men after famine exposure *in utero* and early infancy. *N Engl J Med* 1976; **295**: 349–53

26 Gorski RA, Barraclough CA. Effects of low dosages of androgens on the differentiation of hypothalamic regulatory control of ovulation in the rat. *Endocrinology* 1963; **73**: 210–6

27 Harris G. Sex hormones, brain development and brain function. *Endocrinology* 1964; **75**: 627–48

28 Lorenz K. *Evolution and Modification of Behaviour*. Chicago: University of Chicago Press, 1965

29 Pettitt DJ, Forman MR, Hanson RL, Knowler WC, Bennett PH. Breastfeeding and incidence of non-insulin-dependent diabetes mellitus in Pima Indians. *Lancet* 1997; **350**: 166–8

30 von Kries R, Koletzko B, Sauerwald T *et al*. Breast feeding and obesity: cross sectional study. *BMJ* 1999; **319**: 147–50

31 Hattersley AT, Tooke JE. The fetal insulin hypothesis: an alternative explanation of the association of low birthweight with diabetes and vascular disease. *Lancet* 1999; **353**: 1789–92

32 Fajans SS, Floyd JC, Tattersall RB, Williamson JR, Pek S, Taylor CI. The various faces of diabetes in the young: changing concepts. *Arch Intern Med* 1976; **136**: 194–202

33 Hattersley AT, Beards F, Ballantyne E, Appleton M, Harvey R, Ellard S. Mutations in the

glucokinase gene of the fetus result in reduced birth weight. *Nat Genet* 1998; **19**: 268–70

34 Tamemoto H, Kadowaki T, Tobe K *et al*. Insulin resistance and growth retardation in mice lacking insulin receptor substrate-1. *Nature* 1994; **372**: 182–6

35 Rasmussen SK, Urhammer SA, Hansen T *et al*. Variability of the insulin receptor substrate-1, hepatocyte nuclear factor-1alpha (HNF-1alpha), HNF-4alpha, and HNF-6 genes and size at birth in a population-based sample of young Danish subjects. *J Clin Endocrinol Metab* 2000; **85**: 2951–3

36 McCance DR, Pettitt DJ, Hanson RL, Jacobsson LT, Knowler WC, Bennett PH. Birth weight and non-insulin dependent diabetes: thrifty genotype, thrifty phenotype, or surviving small baby genotype? *BMJ* 1994; **308**: 942–5

37 Pettitt DJ, Knowler WC, Bennett PH, Aleck KA, Baird HR. Obesity in offspring of diabetic Pima Indian women despite normal birth weight. *Diabetes Care* 1987; **10**: 76–80

38 Lindsay RS, Dabelea D, Roumain J, Hanson RL, Bennett PH, Knowler WC. Type 2 diabetes and low birth weight: the role of paternal inheritance in the association of low birth weight and diabetes. *Diabetes* 2000; **49**: 445–9

39 Fall JG, Pulford DJ, Wylie AA, Jirtle RL. Genomic imprinting: implications for human disease. *Am J Pathol* 1999; **154**: 635–47

40 Morison IM, Reeve AE. A catalogue of imprinted genes and parent-of-origin effects in humans and animals. *Hum Mol Genet* 1998; **7**: 1599–609

41 Huxtable SJ, Saker PJ, Haddad L *et al*. Analysis of parent-offspring trios provides evidence for linkage and association between the insulin gene and type 2 diabetes mediated exclusively through paternally transmitted class III variable number tandem repeat alleles. *Diabetes* 2000; **49**: 126–30

42 Poulsen P, Vaag AA, Kyvik KO, Moller JD, Beck-Nielsen H. Low birth weight is associated with NIDDM in discordant monozygotic and dizygotic twin pairs. *Diabetologia* 1997; **40**: 439–46

43 Baird J, Osmond C, MacGregor A, Sneider H, Hales CN, Phillips DIW. Testing the fetal origins hypothesis in twins: the Birmingham twin study. *Diabetologia* 2001; **44**: 33–9

44 Ravelli ACJ, van der Meulen JHP, Michels RPJ, Osmond C, Barker DJP, Hales CN, Bleker OP. Glucose tolerance in adults after prenatal exposure to famine. *Lancet* 1998; **351**: 173–77

45 Lindsay RS, Lindsay RM, Waddell BJ, Seckl JR. Prenatal glucocorticoid exposure leads to offspring hyperglycaemia in the rat: studies with the 11 beta-hydroxysteroid dehydrogenase inhibitor carbenoxolone. *Diabetologia* 1996; **39**: 1299–305

Non-industrialised countries and affluence

Caroline H D Fall

MRC Environmental Epidemiology Unit, University of Southampton, UK

The prevalence of type 2 diabetes is rising rapidly in all non-industrialised populations. By 2025, three-quarters of the world's 300 million adults with diabetes will be in non-industrialised countries, and almost a third in India and China alone. There is strong evidence that this epidemic has been triggered by social and economic development and urbanisation, which are associated with general improvements in nutrition and longevity, but also with obesity, reduced physical exercise and other diabetogenic factors. There is evidence too that fetal growth retardation and growth failure in infancy, both still widespread in non-industrialised populations, increase susceptibility to diabetes. An additional factor may be intergenerational effects of gestational diabetes occurring in mothers who grew poorly in early life and become obese as adults. Prevention of type 2 diabetes will require measures to promote exercise and reduce obesity in adults and children, alongside programmes to achieve healthy fetal and infant growth.

The rising prevalence of type 2 diabetes in non-industrialised populations

Standardised prevalence data for type 2 diabetes are available with a world-wide coverage probably unequalled for any other disease, allowing confident comparisons between people of similar ethnicity living in different settings, and giving a clear picture of secular trends in many populations over the last 20 years. The epidemiological story is remarkably consistent. An epidemic of diabetes is unfolding in countries undergoing rapid economic development and modernisation. Non-industrialised countries are exchanging their high morbidity from infectious disease for morbidity from 'diseases of affluence' including type 2 diabetes and cardiovascular disease.

The prevalence of type 2 diabetes is lowest among people who still have a 'traditional' or 'primitive' lifestyle as either hunter-gatherers or subsistence farmers. Examples are the Mapuche Indians in Chile, rural Bantu in Tanzania, and rural communities in the Pacific islands and South Asia[1–4]. Even in these populations, it cannot be described as a 'rare' disease, affecting 1–3% of people aged 30–64 years. The prevalence is higher in people who have moved away from the traditional way of life,

Correspondence to:
Dr Caroline H D Fall,
MRC Environmental
Epidemiology Unit,
Southampton General
Hospital, Southampton
SO16 6YD, UK

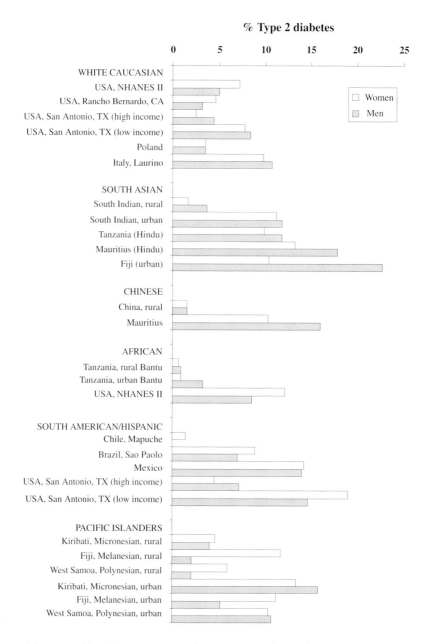

Fig. 1 Prevalence of type 2 diabetes in adults in different ethnic groups and settings (adapted from King & Rewers[1]).

either to live in towns and cities or through migration to another country. This has been described in all major ethnic groups (Fig. 1). Among South Asians, it is less than 5% in rural South India, around 12% in urban South India, and 15–20% in migrants to Mauritius, Fiji, Singapore, Tanzania, The Netherlands and the UK[1,5–12]. Among Chinese, it ranges from less than 3% in rural China to 15–20% in urban Taiwan and Mauritius, and among people of African origin, from less than 3%

in Cameroon, to around 10% among people of West African descent living in Jamaica, and 15% in Jamaicans living in the UK.

The evidence is that high rates of disease in urban centres have arisen within a single generation. The largest increases are described in populations which have undergone the most rapid and extreme change, such as Ethiopian Jews who migrated to Israel, moving from severe malnutrition and a traditional way of life to a modern urban setting. They have a prevalence of 9% compared with 1–2% in Ethiopia itself[13]. Another example is that of the Micronesian Nauruan islanders. Nauru suffered severe deprivation during Japanese occupation in World War II, but became wealthy from phosphate mining post-war[14]. The Nauruans now have one of the highest rates of type 2 diabetes in the world (37% in the 25–74-year-old age group). Examples which may be more typical for large populations in non-industrialised countries, are Mauritius, where the prevalence has increased 30% in Asians, Creoles and Chinese between 1987 and 1998[8], Madras, South India, where it rose by 40% between 1988 and 1994[15], and China, where it is estimated to have increased 3-fold in the last 10 years[16].

Predictions for the future are worse. In 1998, King used the World Health Organization's diabetes database to predict global rates of diabetes for the years 2000 and 2025, based on trends in population size, age structure and urbanisation[17]. According to this analysis, the prevalence will continue to rise, by 30% world-wide, from 4.0% to 5.4%. The number of adults with diabetes will increase from 135 million in 1995 to 300 million in 2025. Although the prevalence will remain higher in industrialised countries, the proportional rise will be greater in non-industrialised countries (48%), and greatest in China (68%) and India (59%). Because of the large populations involved, 75% of the world's adult diabetics will be in non-industrialised countries. India will have more people with diabetes (57 million) than any other country, followed by China (38 million). Unlike industrialised countries, where the highest number of people with diabetes will be in the oldest age groups, in non-industrialised countries this will be in the 45–64 year age group. These predictions agree closely with estimates made by others[18,19].

These estimates apply to type 2 diabetes in adults. An emerging problem, so far reported mainly in native American, African and Hispanic communities in the US, and in Japan, is type 2 diabetes in children and adolescents[20]. Among blacks in Charleston, South Carolina and Hispanics in Ventura, California, 45% of new cases of diabetes in children are type 2. Among Japanese schoolchildren, type 2 diabetes is 7 times more common than type 1, and its incidence has increased 30-fold in the last 20 years. The likelihood is that type 2 diabetes in children will start to emerge in non-industrialised countries too.

The human and economic cost of diabetes

For many people in non-industrialised countries, the cost of even basic treatment for diabetes is crippling[21,22]. Chale estimated annual treatment costs in 1992 at US$287 for those requiring insulin and US$103 for those on oral treatment. Home blood glucose monitoring once a week, which improves diabetic control, costs US$160 per year in Bangladesh[23]. These costs represent 6–12 months' wages for a labourer in the poorest non-industrialised countries. Chale's paper ended with the words: 'if African patients with diabetes have to pay for their treatment most will be unable to do so and will die'. Certainly many patients in poor countries will receive care well below ideal. In a nurse-led community programme in South Africa, home blood glucose monitoring was not available, and not even part of the equation. The target, woefully sub-optimal in modern terms, was simply freedom from symptoms of hyper- or hypo-glycaemia[24].

Good glycaemic control delays the onset of diabetic complications but demands that, in addition to early diagnosis and the availability of drugs and specialist medical care, the patient understands the disease. Poverty and lower levels of education in non-industrialised countries will almost certainly translate into worse disease[25,26]. Many of the large number of people becoming diabetic in middle age will experience its chronic complications during their working lives. Access to treatment for diabetic retinopathy and renal disease, and prosthetic rehabilitation after amputation, are limited. Data from Africa and India show a high prevalence of micro- and macro-albuminuria[27] and a more rapid progression to end-stage renal failure than in Western patients[28]. In the Caribbean countries, a high proportion of surgical cases are patients with diabetic foot problems, and many lower-limb amputees remain permanently bed-ridden because they are not rehabilitated[25]. There are few data from non-industrialised countries on mortality from diabetes, but a report from a tertiary referral centre in Kashmir, India suggested a 10 year reduction in life-span[29]. The commonest causes of death were infection and chronic renal failure, unlike coronary heart disease and stroke, the leading causes of death among people with diabetes in industrialised countries.

Aetiology

Affluence and obesity

The epidemic of type 2 diabetes has been attributed to the 'epidemiological transition', a global trend away from traditional lifestyles and towards urbanisation. In general, urbanisation (and migration) are associated with increased affluence or economic well-being and type 2 diabetes is thought to be a price to pay. This is a complex issue, however. Although early studies in white US and UK populations showed that people with greater affluence, education and social standing had a higher risk of diabetes[30], recent studies show the highest rates of disease in the most deprived sections of the community[31-35]. The same sequence may be repeating itself in non-industrialised countries. Currently, the well-off get more disease[5,16,36]. Type 2 diabetes appears to be a disease of **newly** affluent more than 'established' affluent populations[37]. Consistent with this, while white populations of European origin have moderately high rates of type 2 diabetes (5–10%), which are also rising, their epidemic has been slower and less extreme.

An important feature of the epidemiological transition is obesity. There is a clear association between obesity, which increases insulin resistance, and type 2 diabetes[30]. In all populations, the prevalence of diabetes increases with increasing body mass index. Research from industrialised countries shows that the greater the duration of obesity the higher the risk of diabetes[38,39], and that obesity starting in **childhood** is a risk factor[40]. Therefore, the world-wide trend towards obesity, in both adults and children, is a cause for concern[41-43]. Rates of childhood obesity remain low in some non-industrialised countries such as India (< 1%), but with increasing prosperity have risen to more than 4% in Mauritius, Bolivia and Iran, and more than 10% in Chile and Jamaica[41]. In many non-industrialised populations, this is not perceived as a health problem, indeed quite the opposite. Obesity is often seen as a symbol of health, beauty and status[41,44-46], reflecting a man's ability to provide for his family and a woman's skill as a mother and cook.

Despite its powerful effect on risk, obesity does not fully account for the increase in type 2 diabetes in non-industrialised communities[9,31], where diabetes occurs commonly at levels of body mass index considered healthy in industrialised countries[12,47]. This may be partly explained by the **distribution** of body fat. Central (abdominal) obesity, a characteristic of South Asian populations[48], is more closely linked with type 2 diabetes than generalised or peripheral obesity.

Reduced physical activity

Clinical studies show that exercise increases insulin sensitivity and glucose tolerance[49]. The prevalence of type 2 diabetes is higher in more sedentary people, and individuals with the disease are less active than those without[16,51-53]. Populations with low rates of type 2 diabetes are characterised by the high levels of physical activity associated with hunting and gathering or farming[1,6]. Urbanisation and migration frequently lead to a more sedentary way of life: food and fuel come from shops just down the road, water is on tap and does not have to be carried from the well, there is more labour-saving technology in the home, bicycles are replaced by motorbikes and cars, and work is in offices and factories. Physical activity declines among children too, because of access to television and computer games, and 'hot-house' studying in countries where entry to limited places in higher education is subject to intense competition. Exercise as a healthy leisure activity is a recent Western concept; there are often strong climatic, economic and cultural factors discouraging exercise among urban populations in non-industrialised countries as well as migrants from these countries[44,53].

Poor nutrition: caloric excess and micronutrient deficiency

Himsworth showed reduced mortality and hospital admissions for type 2 diabetes in the UK during periods of wartime food rationing when calorie intakes decreased[54]. Differences in fat intakes correspond well with population differences in the prevalence of type 2 diabetes[31]. On the other hand, prospective studies looking for dietary determinants of diabetes (so far confined to industrialised countries) have failed to show a clear link between carbohydrate or fat intakes and incidence[31,55,56]. Micronutrient deficiency may play a role in susceptibility to disease. Boucher has described an association between vitamin D deficiency and impaired insulin secretion and type 2 diabetes[57]. Although more data are required, there is some evidence too that omega-3 fatty acids, found in green leafy vegetables, nuts, vegetable oils and fish, may protect against a number of cardiovascular risk factors including diabetes[31,58]. Both calorie excess and poor dietary quality are features of urbanisation and migration, especially among the poor, who buy highly refined, energy-dense food, while the better-off can afford a healthier mixed diet[59,60].

Socio-economic inequality and stress

Workers seeking a better life in foreign places often work in menial jobs, have low incomes, live in poor housing, have difficulty communicating, are exposed to crime and aggression, have reduced access to health care and lack traditional family support mechanisms[61]. Associations between social inequality and poor health are well-recognised[62], although poorly understood, and social inequality has been linked to type 2 diabetes and the metabolic syndrome[35]. Possible mechanisms are increased inflammatory cytokines or stimulation of the hypothalamo–pituitary–cortical axis[62].

Environmental toxins

Cassava and other cyanide-containing foods were once thought to be a cause of diabetes in tropical countries. This is not supported by recent evidence, although it remains possible that micronutrient undernutrition or diets low in anti-oxidants, enhance the effects of such environmental toxins[63]. Cities in many non-industrialised countries are chemically polluted, and this has been cited as a possible risk factor for diabetes, acting through the production of inflammatory cytokines[64].

Genes

Finally, the susceptibility to diabetes of populations in non-industrialised countries has been attributed to genes. According to Neel's hypothesis, a 'thrifty genotype' may have enhanced survival in subsistence conditions in the past, but becomes detrimental in a modern urban setting of plentiful food and reduced physical work[65]. Zimmet has proposed that thrifty genes promote fat storage, perhaps mediated by leptin resistance, providing a survival advantage during periods of starvation[6]. It has also been suggested that the tendency to store fat centrally, a feature of South Asian Indian populations, may have a genetic basis. Central body fat, more metabolically active than peripheral fat and less likely to impede locomotion, may have evolved as a site for quick storage and mobilisation in time of need[66]. Though their existence is plausible, these genes have not so far been identified.

Early-life origins of type 2 diabetes

Epidemiological studies in the UK, Europe and the US have shown that men and women who were small at birth, with a low birth weight, are at increased risk of developing cardiovascular disease, hypertension, type 2 diabetes and the metabolic syndrome in adult life[67]. Their findings have led to the 'thrifty phenotype' hypothesis (see elsewhere in this issue) which proposes that fetal undernutrition, occurring at critical periods in the development of pancreatic islet cells and insulin-sensitive tissues such as muscle and liver, has permanent metabolic consequences, including life-long insulin resistance. The epidemiological data suggest that post-natal events modify the risk associated with low birth weight. For example, growth failure in infancy, and the later development of obesity, add to the risk[67].

Intra-uterine growth retardation and failure to thrive in infancy are common in non-industrialised countries, probably largely due to

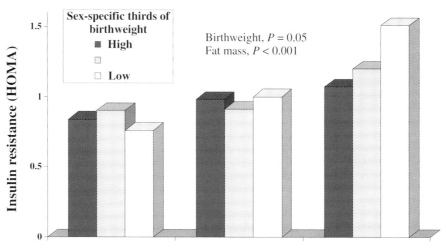

Fig. 2 Insulin resistance (calculated using the HOMA equation) among 8-year-old Indian children (adapted from Bavdekar et al[69]).

maternal stunting and undernutrition. In India, the mean full-term birth weight is 2.6–2.7 kg, almost 1 kg lower than in Western Europe, and 25% of full-term babies are born low birth weight (<2.5 kg)[68]. Most studies linking size at birth with later disease come from industrialised countries, but some data are available from India and China. In India, among children born in the KEM Hospital, Pune, those of lower birth weight were more insulin resistant at the age of 8 years[69]. They showed other features of the metabolic syndrome: higher blood pressure and subscapular/triceps skinfold ratios and lower HDL-cholesterol concentrations. The highest levels of insulin resistance were in children who were small at birth but had a high fat mass at 8 years (Fig. 2). There was a statistically significant interaction between birth weight and 8-year fat mass; the effect of low birth weight was greatest in children with the highest fat mass at 8 years, and the effect of increased 8-year fat mass greatest in children of low birth weight (Fig. 2). Low birth weight was not associated with impaired glucose tolerance at this age, and it is not yet known if insulin resistance in childhood persists into adult life or predicts future diabetes. However, these data suggest that low birth weight leads to insulin resistance when combined with later obesity, and that better intra-uterine growth may protect against the adverse effects of obesity.

Table 1 shows data from studies of young adults in China and India. Among men and women aged 41–47 years born in Beijing, lower birth weight was associated with higher fasting and 2-h plasma glucose and insulin concentrations in an oral glucose tolerance test, and features of the metabolic syndrome including raised systolic blood pressure, higher serum triglyceride concentrations and lower serum HDL-cholesterol

Table 1 2-h plasma glucose concentrations and other components of the insulin resistance syndrome according to birth weight

Birth weight (kg)	n	2-h glucose (mmol/l)	Systolic blood pressure (mmHg)	Serum triglycerides (mmol/l)	Fasting insulin (pmol/l)
Men and women aged 41–47 years in Beijing, China[70]					
≤ 2.5	44	7.9	128	1.77	46
–3.0	184	7.1	125	1.38	47
–3.5	284	6.8	125	1.23	44
> 3.5	115	6.1	122	1.02	33
All	627	6.6	125	1.26	43
P		0.03	0.03	0.008	0.009
Men and women aged 20–45 years in Mysore, South India					
≤ 2.5	58	6.3	121	1.34	35
–3.0	111	6.0	116	1.12	36
–3.5	71	5.4	118	0.98	33
> 3.5	32	5.4	121	0.95	34
All	272	5.8	118	1.10	35
P		0.003	1.0	0.005	0.8

P value adjusted for age, sex, and adult body mass index.
Fall CHD & Veena SR, unpublished data

concentrations[70]. Glucose and insulin concentrations were also inversely related to the mother's body mass index in pregnancy; offspring of thinner mothers were more glucose intolerant and insulin resistant. In a study of young adults (mean age 29 years) born in the Holdsworth Memorial Hospital, Mysore, South India, lower birth weight was associated with higher 2-h glucose concentrations, higher rates of type 2 diabetes and impaired glucose tolerance, and higher serum triglyceride concentrations (Table 1). These findings are similar to those in Western populations and support the 'thrifty phenotype' hypothesis.

A study of older Indian adults (aged 45–65 years) born in Mysore showed somewhat different results[71]. Although lower birth weight subjects had higher fasting insulin concentrations, they did not have higher rates of type 2 diabetes. The prevalence of diabetes was increased in men and women who were short but relatively heavy at birth, with a high ponderal index (birth weight/birth length[3]; Fig. 3A). This group of men and women were characterised by a low 30-min insulin increment, a marker of reduced first phase insulin secretion, even when those with diabetes were excluded (Fig. 3B). There were also surprising associations with maternal weight and pelvimetry; the prevalence of diabetes was increased in offspring of mothers with a higher body weight and larger pelvic intercristal and interspinous external diameters.

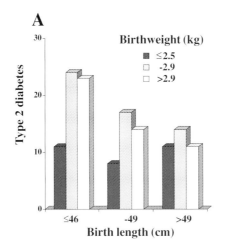
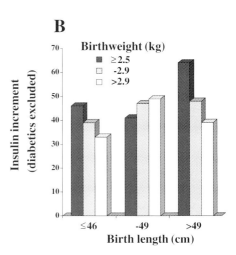

Fig. 3 Prevalence of (A) type 2 diabetes and (B) 30-min insulin increment in men and women born in Mysore, South India[71].

These findings are clearly different from studies in the West and in the younger Pune, Mysore and Beijing cohorts. The link with higher maternal weight and higher ponderal index at birth suggested to us that another factor causing type 2 diabetes in this population may be gestational diabetes, which is associated with maternal obesity and leads to fatter ('macrosomic') babies. In poor communities in India, mothers are often stunted and undernourished, and their babies are born small and thin. According to the 'thrifty phenotype' hypothesis, these babies are at risk of developing insulin resistance in childhood and adult life, especially if their circumstances in later life allow them to become obese. If they are female, their insulin resistance will be further exacerbated in pregnancy, and may lead to gestational diabetes. There is a growing evidence that women who experienced deprivation in early life, indicated by low birth weight[72–75] and/or short stature[76–78] have an increased risk of developing this complication of pregnancy.

Effects of maternal gestational diabetes

It is well-established that the offspring of mothers with diabetes in pregnancy are at increased risk of developing adult type 2 diabetes. This has been most clearly shown among the US Pima Indians, who have high rates of gestational diabetes (Fig. 4A)[79], and recently confirmed in white Caucasians in the US Nurse's Study[80]. Among the Pima Indians, 70% of people with prenatal exposure to a diabetic environment were diabetic at 25–34 years of age (Fig. 4A)[79]. This phenomenon is probably environmentally rather than genetically mediated; mothers who were prediabetic, and developed diabetes at some time **after** their pregnancy,

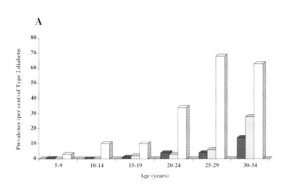
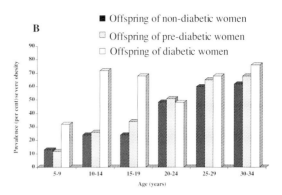

A

B
■ Offspring of non-diabetic women
□ Offspring of pre-diabetic women
□ Offspring of diabetic women

Fig. 4 Prevalence of (A) type 2 diabetes and (B) severe obesity in offspring of non-diabetic, prediabetic and diabetic women: data from the Pima Indians[79].

did not transmit this high risk to their offspring (Fig. 4A). This is supported by animal studies in which induction of diabetes or hyperglycaemia in mother rats using streptozotocin or glucose infusion leads to insulin resistance, deficits in insulin secretion, and diabetes in the offspring[81,82].

The importance of gestational diabetes as a factor in the epidemic of type 2 diabetes in non-industrialised countries is not known, and there are few recent data on the incidence of gestational diabetes. In her world-wide review, King cites low rates of 3.5% in Karachi, Pakistan, 0.6% in Madras, India and 0.6% in Taipei, China[83]. A recent prospective study in Mysore, India, however, showed a much higher incidence of 6%[78]. The babies born in this study are being followed up to determine the effects on their glucose/insulin metabolism. Rates of gestational diabetes are known to be high among women from non-industrialised countries who have migrated to more affluent countries. In Melbourne, Australia, the prevalence was 15% among Asian women, 14% among Chinese and 10% among women of African origin, compared with only 5% among white Caucasian women. Similarly, in London, UK, 6% of Asian mothers and 3% of Afro-Caribbean mothers developed gestational diabetes compared with 1% of white Caucasian women[83]. It seems likely that gestational diabetes is playing a role in fuelling the rise in type 2 diabetes that occurs with the epidemiological transition in non-industrialised countries. Figure 5 presents a model to explain how increasing prosperity and urbanisation, in populations made insulin resistant by generations of fetal malnutrition, leads to the appearance of gestational diabetes and a rising epidemic of type 2 diabetes.

Both intra-uterine undernutrition and maternal diabetes may lead to obesity and hence increased risk of type 2 diabetes. Boys exposed *in utero* to the Dutch famine were at increased risk of obesity in early adult life[84]. Low birth weight has been shown to be associated with central

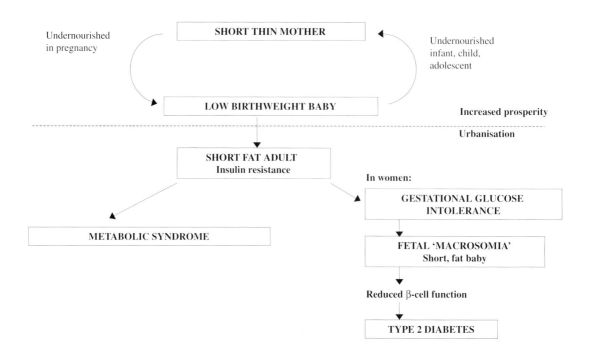

Fig. 5 Proposed intergenerational effects of intra-uterine growth retardation and gestational diabetes in causing type 2 diabetes in non-industrialised countries (adapted from Fall *et al*[71]).

obesity in studies of adults and children in the UK and India[69,85]. At birth, Indian babies are lighter than UK babies, but have similar amounts of truncal body fat, measured by subscapular skinfold thickness, suggesting fat preservation despite growth retardation[86,87]. It is not yet known whether this persists post-natally. The Pima Indian studies have shown that maternal gestational diabetes is also associated with a high risk of obesity in the next generation, especially in childhood and young adult life (Fig. 4B)[79].

Prevention of type 2 diabetes

Despite clearly identified modifiable environmental risk factors for type 2 diabetes, surprisingly little is done about its prevention in Western countries compared, for example, with coronary heart disease. This may be because relatively few people develop diabetes, those who do can generally afford to be treated, and major complications tend to develop only late in life. If the predictions hold true, however, and prevalence rates of 10–20% become typical in urban communities in non-industrialised countries, the situation will be very different and impossible to ignore. Preventive measures are urgently needed.

Among US Hispanics and Japanese, the high prevalence of type 2 diabetes compared with white Caucasians is most marked in people of low education[32,33]. Despite its association with higher income and socio-economic status, studies from non-industrialised countries have also identified lack of education as a risk factor for diabetes[16,88]. Stern has predicted a 'descending limb' to epidemics of the disease, as people become better educated, learn to eat better, avoid obesity and lead more active lives[32]. In an important and so far unique test of this, Pan conducted a randomised, controlled trial of diet and/or exercise in men and women with impaired glucose tolerance living in Da Qing, China[89]. Subjects were identified by screening 110,660 people, and randomised by centre to receive advice on diet, exercise, both or neither (control group). Dietary advice included detailed recommendations about intakes of carbohydrate, fat, protein, vegetables and alcohol and achieving a target body mass index. People in the exercise groups were advised to increase their activity by at least one 'unit' per day (30 min of slow walking, 20 min of fast walking, 10 min of strenuous exercise (*e.g.* running) or 5 min of very strenuous exercise (*e.g.* swimming or skipping). Advice was given one-to-one by a physician, and later in groups, and continued regularly for 6 years of follow-up.

During 6 years, the incidence of diabetes was 68% in the control group, but significantly lower (40–50%) in all three intervention groups (Fig. 6A), despite no effect on mean body mass index (Fig. 6B). Dietary advice was as

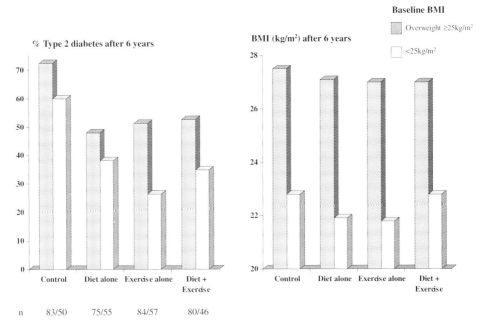

Fig. 6 Effect of diet and exercise in preventing type 2 diabetes in a randomised, controlled trial among people with impaired glucose tolerance in Da Qing, China[89].

effective as exercise, and there was no apparent benefit of combining the two. The subjects, most of whom migrated to Da Qing from all over China to work in the oil industry are probably representative of many populations undergoing the epidemiological transition in the non-industrialised world. This study is important in showing that intervention is possible and effective, though potentially expensive on a large scale. It needs to be replicated, and further studies are needed to determine whether primary intervention, when glucose tolerance is still normal, or in childhood, is effective. Enough is known, however, to recommend strongly the promotion of exercise and avoidance of obesity in non-industrialised populations.

The 'thrifty phenotype' hypothesis would predict that diabetes will recede naturally when nutrition improves sufficiently and for enough time (probably at least one generation) to lead to improvements in fetal nutrition and growth. That this could happen is supported by animal experiments. Sand rats transferred from a wild to a caged environment become obese and diabetic[90]. The effects are worst in the generation directly transferred and become milder, then disappear, in subsequent generations. So far, there has been only one report of a fall in the incidence of diabetes in a human population, the Nauruan islanders[14]. Their age-specific prevalence fell from 28% in 1975/1976 to 24% in 1987, despite no reduction in obesity or increase in physical activity. The authors of this report suggested that the decline was due to reduced fertility in women with a strong genetic tendency for and, therefore early onset of, type 2 diabetes. An alternative explanation is that prosperity has led to improved fetal nutrition and thus to individuals who are less susceptible to diabetes.

The potential to prevent type 2 diabetes can been added to a long list of reasons to recommend the promotion of healthy fetal and infant growth in non-industrialised countries. There are large gaps in scientific knowledge as to the best ways of achieving this. Enough is known, however, to recommend improvements in the nutrition and growth of (female) infants, children and adolescents, encouraging the delaying of childbearing until the mother's own growth is complete, and promoting adequate maternal intakes of energy, protein and micronutrients during pregnancy itself[87,91–93]. There is sufficient evidence of long-term adverse effects of gestational diabetes on the offspring to recommend that in populations with adequate energy intakes mothers, especially those who are stunted and at increased risk of gestational diabetes, should avoid becoming obese. Finally, screening for and intensive management of gestational diabetes should probably become more rigorous.

Acknowledgements

I would like to thank my colleagues and collaborators in India, especially Drs AN Pandit, CS Yajnik (KEM Hospital, Pune), S Rao (Agharkar Research

Institute, Pune), BDR Paul, L David, CE Stein, JC Hill, K Kumaran and SR Veena (Holdsworth Memorial Hospital, Mysore), and the following funding agencies which have supported my research there: the Medical Research Council, the Wellcome Trust, the Parthenon Trust, the Department for International Development and the Wessex Medical Trust.

References

1   King H, Rewers M. Global estimates for prevalence of diabetes mellitus and impaired glucose tolerance in adults. *Diabetes Care* 1993: **16**: 157–77
2   Swai ABM, McLarty DG, Kitange HM *et al*. Low prevalence of risk factors for coronary heart disease in rural Tanzania. *Int J Epidemiol* 1993; **22**: 651–9
3   Cooper RS, Forrester T, Rotimi CN *et al*. Prevalence of NIDDM among populations of the African diaspora. *Diabetes Care* 1997; **20**: 343–8
4   Ramachandran A, Dharmaraj D, Snehalatha C, Viswanathan M. Prevalence of glucose intolerance in Asian Indians; urban-rural difference and significance of upper body adiposity. *Diabetes Care* 1992; **15**: 1348–55
5   Ramachandran A, Jali MV, Mohan V, Snehalatha C, Viswanathan M. High prevalence of diabetes in an urban population in south India. *BMJ* 1988; **297**: 587–90
6   Zimmet PZ, McCarty DJ, de Courten MP. The global epidemiology of non-insulin-dependent diabetes mellitus and the metabolic syndrome. *J Diabetes Complications* 1997; **11**: 60–8
7   Middelkoop BJ, Kesarlal-Sadhoeram SM, Ramsaransing GN, Struben HW. Diabetes mellitus among South Asian inhabitants of The Hague: high prevalence and age-specific socio-economic gradient. *Int J Epidemiol* 1999; **28**: 1119–23
8   Zimmet P. Globalization, coca-colonization and the chronic disease epidemic: can the Doomsday scenario be averted? *J Intern Med* 2000; **247**: 301–10
9   Mbanya J-CN, Cruickshank JK, Forrester T *et al*. Standardised comparison of glucose intolerance in West African-origin populations of rural and urban Cameroon, Jamaica, and Caribbean migrants to Britain. *Diabetes Care* 1999; **22**: 434–40
10 Unwin N, Alberti KGMM, Bhopal R, Harland J, Watson W, White M. Comparison of the current WHO and new ADA criteria for the diagnosis of diabetes mellitus in three ethnic groups in the UK. *Diabet Med* 1998; **15**: 554–7
11 McKeigue PM, Miller GJ, Marmot MG. Coronary heart disease in South Asians overseas: a review. *J Clin Epidemiol* 1989; **42**: 597–609
12 Chen KT, Chen CJ, Gregg EW, Williamson DF, Narayan KMV. High prevalence of impaired fasting glucose and type 2 diabetes mellitus in Penghu islets, Taiwan: evidence of a rapidly emerging epidemic? *Diabetes Res Clin Pract* 1999; **44**: 56–69
13 Cohen MP, Stern E, Rusecki Y, Zeidler A. High prevalence of diabetes in young adult Ethiopian immigrants to Israel. *Diabetes* 1988; **37**: 824–8
14 Dowse GK, Zimmet PZ, Finch CF, Collins VR. Decline in incidence of epidemic glucose intolerance in Nauruans: implications for the 'thrifty genotype'. *Am J Epidemiol* 1991; **133**: 1093–104
15 Ramachandran A, Snehalatha C, Latha E, Vijay V, Viswanathan M. Rising prevalence of NIDDM in an urban population in India. *Diabetologia* 1997; **40**: 232–7
16 Pan X-R, Liu J, Yang W-Y, Li G-W. Prevalence of diabetes and its risk factors in China, 1994. *Diabetes Care* 1997; **20**: 1664–9
17 King H, Aubert RE, Herman WH. Global burden of diabetes, 1995–2025; prevalence, numerical estimates and projections. *Diabetes Care* 1998; **21**: 1414–31
18 Amos AF, McCarty DJ, Zimmet P. The rising global burden of diabetes and its complications: estimates and projections to the year 2010. *Diabet Med* 1997; **14** (**Suppl 5**): S7–85
19 Murray CJL, Lopez AD. *Global Health Statistics: Global Burden of Disease and Injury Series*, vol II. Boston, MA: Harvard School of Public Health, 1996
20 American Diabetes Association. Type 2 diabetes in children and adolescents. *Pediatrics* 2000; **105**: 671–80

21 Chale SS, Swai ABM, Mujinja PGM, McLarty DG. Must diabetes be a fatal disease in Africa? Study of the costs of treatment. *BMJ* 1992; **304**: 1215–8

22 Shobana R, Rama Rao P, Lavanya A, Williams R, Vijay V, Ramachandran A. Expenditure on health care incurred by diabetic subjects in a developing country – a study from South India. *Diabetes Res Clin Pract* 2000; **48**: 37-42

23 Kibriya MG, Ali L, Banik NG, Azad Khan AK. Home monitoring of blood glucose (HMBG) in Type 2 diabetes mellitus in a developing country. *Diabetes Res Clin Pract* 1999; **46**: 253–7

24 Coleman R, Gill G, Wilkinson D. Non-communicable disease management in resource-poor settings: a primary care model from rural South Africa. *Bull World Health Organ* 1998; **76**: 633–40

25 Gulliford MC. Controlling non-insulin-dependent diabetes mellitus in developing countries. *Int J Epidemiol* 1995; **24** (**Suppl 1**): S53–9

26 Famuyiwa OO. Important considerations in the care of diabetic patients in a developing country (Nigeria). *Diabet Med* 1990; **7**: 927–30

27 Rahlenbeck SI, Gebre-Yohannes A. Prevalence and epidemiology of micro- and macroalbumimuria in Ethiopian diabetic patients. *J Diabetes Complications* 1997; **11**: 343–9

28 Chugh KS, Kumar R, Sakhuja V, Pereira BJG, Gupta A. Nephropathy in type 2 diabetes mellitus in third world countries – Chandigarh Study. *Int J Artif Organs* 1989; **12**: 299–302

29 Zargar AH, Wani AI, Masoodi SH, Laway BA, Bashir MI. Mortality in diabetes mellitus – data from a developing region of the world. *Diabetes Res Clin Pract* 1999; **43**: 67–74

30 West KM. *Epidemiology of Diabetes and its Vascular Lesions*. New York: Elsevier, 1978

31 Hamman RF. Genetic and environmental determinants of non-insulin-dependent diabetes mellitus (NIDDM). *Diabetes Metab Rev* 1992; **8**: 287–338

32 Stern MP, Knapp JA, Hazuda HP, Haffner SM, Patterson JK, Mitchell BD. Genetic and environmental determinants of type II diabetes in Mexican Americans; is there a 'descending limb' to the modernisation/diabetes relationship? *Diabetes Care* 1991; **14** (**Suppl 3**): 649–54

33 Leonetti DL, Tsunehara CH, Wahl PW, Fujimoto WY. Educational achievement and the risk of non-insulin-dependent diabetes or coronary heart disease in Japanese-American men. *Ethn Dis* 1992; **2**: 326–36

34 Meadows P. Variations of diabetes mellitus prevalence in general practice and its relation to deprivation. *Diabet Med* 1995; **12**: 696–700

35 Brunner EJ, Marmot M, Nanchahal K *et al*. Social inequality in coronary risk: central obesity and the metabolic syndrome. Evidence from the Whitehall II Study. *Diabetologia* 1997; **40**: 1341–9

36 Herman WH, Ali MA, Engelou MM, Kenny SY, Gunter EM, Malarcher AM. Diabetes mellitus in Egypt: risk factors and prevalence. *Diabet Med* 1995; **12**: 1126-31.

37 Morris JA. Fetal origin of maturity-onset diabetes mellitus: genetic or environmental cause? *Med Hypotheses* 1997; **51**: 285–8

38 Everhart JE, Pettitt DJ, Bennett PH, Knowler WC. Duration of obesity increases the incidence of NIDDM. *Diabetes* 1992; **41**: 235–40

39 Wannamethee SG, Shaper AG. Weight change and duration of overweight and obesity in the incidence of Type 2 diabetes. *Diabetes Care* 1999; **22**: 1266–72

40 Vanhala M, Vanhala P, Kumpusalo E, Halonen P, Takala J. Relation between obesity from childhood to adulthood and the metabolic syndrome: population based study. *BMJ* 1998; **317**: 319

41 Shetty PS. Obesity in children in developing countries: indicator of economic progress or a prelude to a health disaster. *Indian Pediatr* 1999; **36**: 11–5

42 Drewnowski A, Popkin BM. The nutrition transition: new trends in global diet. *Nutr Rev* 1997; **55**: 31–43

43 Popkin BM, Richards MK, Montiero CA. Stunting is associated with overweight in children of four nations who are undergoing the nutrition transition. *J Nutr* 1996; **126**: 3009–16

44 Carter-Nolan PL, Adams-Campbell LL, Williams J. Recruitment strategies for black women at risk for non-insulin-dependent diabetes mellitus into exercise protocols: a qualitative assessment. *J Natl Med Assoc* 1996; **88**: 558–62

45 Hoyos MD, Clarke H. Concepts of obesity in family practice. *West Indian Med J* 1987; **36**: 95–8

46 Coughlan A, McCarty DJ, Jorgensen LN, Zimmet P. The epidemic of NIDDM in Asian and Pacific Island populations: prevalence and risk factors. *Horm Metab Res* 1997; **29**: 323–31

47 Seidell JC. Obesity, insulin resistance and diabetes – a worldwide epidemic. *Br J Nutr* 2000; **83 (Suppl 1)**: S5–8

48 Shelgikar GM, Hockaday TDR, Yajnik CS. Central rather than generalised obesity is related to hyperglycaemia in Asian Indian subjects. *Diabet Med* 1991; **8**: 712–7

49 Boughouts LB, Keizer HA. Exercise and insulin sensitivity: a review. *Int J Sports Med* 2000; **21**: 1–12

50 Manson JE, Rimm EB, Stampfer MJ *et al.* Physical activity and incidence of non-insulin-dependent diabetes mellitus in women. *Lancet* 1991; **338**: 774–8

51 Levitt NS, Steyns K, Lambert EV *et al.* Modifiable risk factors for type 2 diabetes mellitus in a peri-urban community in South Africa. *Diabet Med* 1999; **16**: 946–50

52 Zimmet PZ, Collins VR, Dowse GK *et al.* The relation of physical activity to cardiovascular risk factors in Mauritians. *Am J Epidemiol* 1991; **134**: 862–75

53 Dhawan J, Bray CL, Warburton R, Ghambhir DS, Morris J. Insulin resistance, high prevalence of diabetes, and cardiovascular risk in immigrant Asians. Genetic or environmental effect? *Br Heart J* 1994; **72**: 413–21

54 Himsworth HP. Diet and the incidence of diabetes mellitus. *Clin Sci* 1935; **2**: 117–48

55 Lundgren H, Bengtsson C, Blohme G *et al.* Dietary habits and incidence of non-insulin-dependent diabetes mellitus in a population study of women in Gothenburg, Sweden. *Am J Clin Nutr* 1989; **49**: 708–12

56 Colditz GA, Manson JE, Stampfer MJ, Rosner B, Willett WC, Speizer FE. Diet and risk of clinical diabetes in women. *Am J Clin Nutr* 1992; **55**: 1018–23

57 Boucher BJ. Inadequate vitamin D status: does it contribute to the disorders comprising syndrome X? *Br J Nutr* 1998; **79**: 315–27

58 Raheja BS. Diabetes and atherosclerosis as immune inflammatory disorders: options for reversal of disease processes. *J Assoc Physicians India* 1994; **42**: 385–90

59 Popkin BM, Keyou G, Fengying Z, Guo X, Haijiang M, Zohoori N. The nutrition transition in China: a cross-sectional analysis. *Eur J Clin Nutr* 1993; **47**: 333–46

60 McDermott R. Ethics, epidemiology and the thrifty gene: biological determinism is a health hazard. *Soc Sci Med* 1998; **47**: 1189–95

61 Greenhalgh PM. Diabetes in British South Asians: nature, nurture, and culture. *Diabet Med* 1997; **14**: 10–8

62 Marmot M. Epidemiology of socio-economic status and health: are determinants within countries the same as between countries. *Ann N Y Acad Sci* 1999; **896**: 16–29

63 Harsha Rao B, Yajnik CS. Commentary: time to rethink malnutrition and diabetes in the tropics. *Diabetes Care* 1996; **19**: 1014–7

64 Yudkin JS, Yajnik CS, Mohamed-Ali V, Bulmer K. High levels of circulating pro-inflammatory cytokines and leptin in urban but not rural Indians. *Diabetes Care* 1999; **22**: 363–4

65 Neel JV. Diabetes mellitus: a 'thrifty' genotype rendered detrimental by 'progress'? *Am J Hum Genet* 1962; **14**: 353–62

66 McKeigue PM, Keen H. Diabetes, insulin, ethnicity and coronary heart disease. In: Marmot M, Elliott P. (eds) *Coronary Heart Disease Epidemiology; from Aetiology to Public Health.* Oxford: Oxford Medical Publications, 1992

67 Barker DJP. *Mothers, Babies and Disease in Later Life.* London: BMJ Publishing Group, 1994

68 Sachdev HPS. Low birth weight in South Asia. In: Gillespie S. (ed) *Malnutrition in South Asia; a Regional Profile.* South Asia: UNICEF, 1997; 23–50

69 Bavdekar A, Yajnik CS, Fall CHD *et al.* The insulin resistance syndrome (IRS) in eight-year-old Indian children: small at birth, big at 8 years or both? *Diabetes* 2000; **48**: 2422–9

70 Jie Mi, Law C, Zhang Khong-Lai, Osmond C, Stein C, Barker D. Effects of infant birthweight and maternal body mass index in pregnancy on components of the insulin resistance syndrome in China. *Ann Intern Med* 2000; **132**: 253–60

71 Fall CHD, Stein C, Kumaran K *et al.* Size at birth, maternal weight, and non-insulin-dependent diabetes (NIDDM) in South Indian adults. *Diabet Med* 1998; **15**: 220–7

72 Olah KS. Low maternal birthweight – an association with impaired glucose tolerance in pregnancy. *J Obstet Gynaecol* 1996; **16**: 5–8

73 Plante LA. Small size at birth and later diabetic pregnancy. *Obstet Gynecol* 1998; **92**: 781–4

74 Williams MA, Emanuel I, Kimpo C, Leisenring M, Hale CB. A population-based cohort study of the relation between maternal birthweight and risk of gestational diabetes mellitus in four racial/ethnic groups. *Paediatr Perinat Epidemiol* 1999; **13**: 452–65

75 Egeland GM, Skaerven R, Irgens LM. Birth characteristics of women who develop gestational diabetes: population based study. *BMJ* 2000; **321**: 546–7

76 Anastasiou E, Alevizaki M, Grigorakis SSJ, Phillippou G, Kyprianou M, Souvatzoglou A. Decreased stature in gestational diabetes mellitus. *Diabetologia* 1998; **41**: 997–1001

77 Jang HC, Min HK, Lee HK, Cho N, Metzger BE. Short stature in Korean women: a contribution to the multifactorial predisposition to gestational diabetes mellitus. *Diabetologia* 1998; **41**: 778–83

78 Hill JC, Krishnaveni GV, Fall CHD, Kellingray SD. Glucose tolerance and insulin status during pregnancy in South India: relationships to maternal and neonatal body composition. *J Endocrinol* 2000; **164** (**Suppl**): P252

79 Dabelea D, Knowler WC, Pettitt DJ. Effect of diabetes in pregnancy on offspring: follow-up research in the Pima Indians. *J Matern-Fetal Med* 2000; **9**: 83–8

80 Rich-Edwards J, Colditz G, Stampfer M *et al*. Birthweight and the risk for type 2 diabetes mellitus in adult women. *Ann Intern Med* 1999; **130**: 278–84

81 Bihoreau MT, Ktorza A, Kinebanyan MF, Picon L. Impaired glucose homeostasis in adult rats from hyperglycaemic mothers. *Diabetes* 1986; **35**: 979–84

82 Aerts L, Holemans K, Van Assche FA. Maternal diabetes during pregnancy: consequences for the offspring. *Diabetes Metab Rev* 1990; **6**: 147–67

83 King H. Epidemiology of glucose intolerance and gestational diabetes in women of childbearing age. *Diabetes Care* 1998; **21** (**Suppl 2**): B9–13

84 Ravelli GP, Stein ZA, Susser MW. Obesity in young men after famine exposure *in utero* and early infancy. *N Engl J Med* 1976; **295**: 349–53

85 Law CM, Barker DJP, Osmond C, Fall CHD, Simmonds SJ. Early growth and abdominal fatness in adult life. *J Epidemiol Community Health* 1992; **46**: 184–6

86 Yajnik CS. The insulin resistance epidemic in India: small at birth, big as adult? *IDF Bull* 1998; **43**: 23–8

87 Fall CHD, Yajnik CS, Rao S, Coyaji KJ. Effects of maternal body composition on fetal growth; the Pune Maternal Nutrition and Fetal Growth Study. In: O'Brien PMS, Wheeler T, Barker DJP. (eds) *Fetal Programming; Influences on Development and Disease in Later Life*. London: RCOG Press, 1999

88 Al-Mahroos F, Al-Roomi K, McKeigue PM. Relation of high blood pressure to glucose intolerance, plasma lipids and educational status in an Arabian Gulf population. *Int J Epidemiol* 2000; **29**: 71–6

89 Pan X-R, Cao H-B, Li G-W *et al*. Effects of diet and exercise in preventing NIDDM in people with impaired glucose tolerance; the Da Qing IGT and Diabetes Study. *Diabetes Care* 1997; **20**: 537–44

90 Renold AE, Stauffacher W, Cahill GF. Diabetes mellitus In: Stanbury H. (ed) *The Metabolic Basis of Inherited Disease*. New York: McGraw-Hill, 1972

91 Kramer MS. Determinants of low birthweight: methodological assessment and meta-analysis. *Bull World Health Organ* 1987; **65**: 663–737

92 Ceesay SM, Prentice AM, Cole TM *et al*. Effects on birthweight and perinatal mortality of maternal dietary supplements in rural Gambia: 5 year randomised controlled trial. *BMJ* 1997; **315**: 786–90

93 Rao S, Yajnik CS, Kanade A, Fall CHD, Margetts BM, Jackson AA *et al*. Intake of micronutrient-rich foods in rural Indian mothers is associated with the size of their babies at birth. The Pune Maternal Nutrition Study. *J Nutr* 2001; 131: 1217–24

Obesity and its potential mechanistic basis

Andrew M Prentice

MRC International Nutrition Group, London School of Hygiene and Tropical Medicine, London, UK and MRC Keneba, The Gambia

Obesity plays a central role in the development of the thrifty phenotype. The metabolic disturbances of the cardiovascular metabolic syndrome, frequently ascribed to the thrifty phenotype, are rare in the absence of obesity and their expression is generally proportional to the size of the excess fat mass. Thus obesity interacts with early-life programming in the establishment of disease. Surprisingly, the evidence that fetal or infant diet leads to programming of obesity itself is rather weak, though this may be explained by the fact that life-style influences obscure the linkage between metabolic predisposition and maturity-onset obesity. This paper summarises the possible metabolic basis of obesity with special reference to those processes for which there are plausible mechanisms by which long-term programming may operate. It is concluded that the newly-emerging molecular discoveries in body weight regulatory systems point to the need for detailed studies of gene–environment interactions and life-course influences before we will fully understand the aetiology of complex phenotypes such as the metabolic syndrome.

There is a rapidly emerging pandemic of obesity in affluent nations[1]. This is of central importance to the topic of this issue, the thrifty phenotype, since it creates the conditions in which the metabolic disturbances programmed by early-life events find their fullest expression. Obesity seems to play both a permissive role in the emergence of the thrifty phenotype (the metabolic syndrome is rare in the absence of obesity) and an active role (there is a dose-dependent relationship between the level of obesity and its pathological sequelae).

Rather surprisingly, there seems less evidence that the development of obesity is itself a manifestation of a thrifty phenotype, at least in regard to the effects of fetal and early-life programming which are less strong in terms of adiposity than might be expected given the evidence for other metabolic changes[2–4]. This observation might be explained by the fact that obesity is a highly multifactorial syndrome in which social, behavioural and environmental influences might over-ride some of the underlying metabolic pressures entrained as part of the thrifty phenotype.

Correspondence to: Prof. Andrew M Prentice, MRC International Nutrition Group, Public Health Nutrition Unit, London School of Hygiene and Tropical Medicine, 49–51 Bedford Square, London WC1B 3DP, UK

Obesity – a complex multifactorial disease

The sharp increase in obesity rates in the late 20th century has been a readily predictable outcome of the major environmental transition that has created an abundant food supply and sedentary life-styles[5]. However, the factors that determine which individuals are most susceptible to the external effects of this new environment are more complex. The schematic in Figure 1 illustrates the interplay of the various factors influencing a person's tendency to gain weight. The innate physiological and metabolic processes regulating energy balance lie at the centre. The blueprint for these is genetically encoded. In rare instances, there are single major gene defects which cause obesity (*see below*). More commonly, obesity arises in individuals who carry a cluster of genes each of which creates only a minor tendency towards energy accretion, but whose combined effects can lead to a pronounced weight gain in an appropriate environmental setting. The term 'thrifty genotype', first coined by Neel in the 1960s, has been widely used to encapsulate the notion of a gene, or set of genes, which assist their carriers to lay down energy more rapidly in times of feasting and to conserve their energy usage during times of famine, thus conferring survival value[6]. The identity of these thrifty genes has proved elusive, but

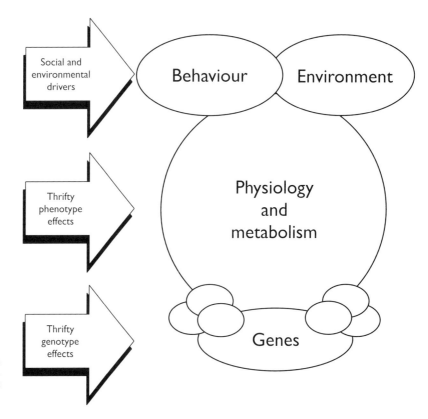

Fig 1 Multifactorial interactions influencing the development of obesity.

the general concept remains useful and it can be demonstrated that famine has been an ever-present selective pressure on human populations and may lie at the origins of modern-day obesity[7].

The readout from the genetic blueprint (*i.e.* the translation of genotype to phenotype) can be permanently modified by an individual's fetal and early-life experiences particularly in regard of placental nutrient supply and infant feeding. Examples of this are known for individual substrates. For instance, baboons that were breast-fed or formula-fed in infancy show altered cholesterol metabolism and lipoprotein levels as adults[8]. The concept of the 'thrifty phenotype' first developed by Hales and Barker[9] extends this idea to suggest that a general shortage of energy-supplying fuels in early life may create a metabolism which is permanently programmed to expect a frugal food supply and, therefore, has difficulty in coping with abundance. In this respect, the thrifty phenotype is analogous to Neel's thrifty genotype[6] – a useful adaptation which has been 'rendered detrimental by progress'.

In a single generation, the levels of obesity in affluent countries have altered so radically as to require a major overhaul of our explanatory paradigms. In Figure 2, the hatched bars illustrate the approximate population distribution of body mass index (BMI) in the UK some 30 years ago. Under such circumstances, any individual exceeding the clinical threshold for obesity (≥ 30 kg/m^2) would have been at the extreme right-hand end of the distribution and it was highly likely that they carried a pronounced

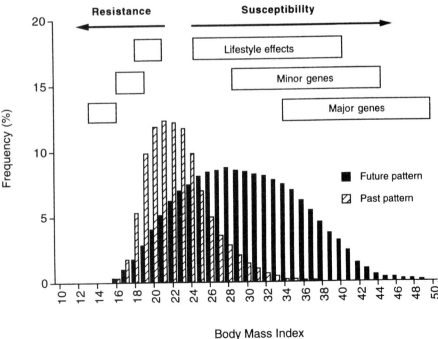

Fig 2 Secular changes in the balance of factors influencing obesity.

genetic propensity towards fat gain. However, the current and projected distributions (solid bars) are shifted substantially to the right by the increasing prevalence of 'life-style' obesity. Under such circumstances, it becomes much more difficult to detect true genetic and metabolic susceptibility. As obesity rates climb still further, the whole concept of genetic susceptibility increasingly loses validity, and as obesity becomes the norm it becomes more interesting to examine evidence for genetic resistance to obesity. It is possible that a similar general argument could explain the relatively weak evidence linking early-life events to later obesity; any underlying association might be obscured by the over-whelming lifestyle influences.

Genetic factors

The very rapid increase in obesity in populations in which there has been a minimal infusion of new genes through immigration and inter-marriage provides unequivocal proof of the importance of environmental factors. This, however, does not diminish the importance of understanding genetic susceptibility to obesity. Indeed, it is work in the latter domain that has recently provided a quantum leap in our knowledge of the mechanistic basis of obesity.

Monogenic disorders

Certain discrete (probably monogenic) disorders in which severe obesity is one part of a pleiotropic clinical picture have been known for many years (*e.g.* Prader-Willi and Bardet-Biedl syndromes)[10]. In such cases, the obesity is usually viewed as just one of many symptoms and usually has a clear aetiology, as in the case of the voracious and seemingly unquenchable appetite typical of the Prader-Willi patient. More recently, there has been a series of discoveries of monogenic mutations in which obesity appears to be one of the most prominent aspects of the symptomatology and was the basis of the initial genetic screening for mutations[11]. Several of these new Mendelian causes of human obesity appear to be directly homologous to mouse mutations that have been known and studied for decades, thus providing additional insight into the biology underlying the effects of each mutation (*see* Table 1). A recent *Nature Insight* publication provides an excellent series of reviews for readers interested in a detailed coverage of these new genetic discoveries and of the understanding they provide about the regulation of energy balance[12]. In the present context, a brief description of two of these mutations will suffice to put the monogenic disorders into perspective in relation to the overall problem of obesity.

Table 1 A selection of genetic mutations causing homologous obesity in mice and humans

Mutation	Mechanism
obese	Absence of functional circulating leptin leads to absence of feed-back signal from adipose tissue stores
diabetes	Loss of function of leptin receptor in hypothalamus
fat	Loss of function of carboxypeptidase E responsible for processing receptors for endocrine and neuroendocrine prohormones
MC4r	Loss of function of brain receptor for α-MSH and agouti-related protein
POMC	Loss of function of precursor of brain α-MSH and β-endorphin
A^y	Ectopic expression of agouti protein: antagonist of melanocortin receptors

Cited in Barsh et al[11].

In 1994, Friedman and colleagues used positional cloning to identify the gene defect responsible for the severe obesity of the *ob/ob* mouse[13]. The gene encodes an adipocyte-derived hormone, leptin, which is secreted into the circulation in proportion to the size of the adipose tissue mass. Leptin crosses the blood–brain barrier and signals to the central nervous system through leptin receptors in the arcuate nucleus of the hypothalamus[14]. In the *db/db* mouse, obesity is caused by a mutation leading to non-functioning leptin receptors[15]. The circulating plasma leptin signal correlates both with the size of the adipocytes and with their energy flux. It thus provides the brain with a very effective fuel gauge that integrates information on both the long-term and short-term energy status of peripheral tissues. A complex series of neural circuits activated by leptin act to modulate appetite, energy expenditure (at least in mice), reproductive function and immunity (again in mice)[14,16]. This energy regulating system is sometimes termed an 'adipostat'.

Human homologues with defects in leptin and in the leptin receptor have now been traced but are extremely rare, having been identified in just a handful of in-bred families throughout the world[11,17]. Nonetheless, these discoveries provide unparalleled insight into the biology of body weight regulation by showing that a defect in either the signal or the receptor can lead to increased appetite and subsequent hyperphagia leading to morbid obesity. In leptin-deficient patients, substitution of the defective natural leptin by regular injection of human recombinant leptin has also been shown to suppress appetite and lead to impressive weight loss[18]. Other cases of human obesity arise from mutations involving some of the signalling steps downstream of leptin, but all are extremely rare. In spite of a world-wide search for such mutations by numerous research teams, there were only 22 individuals affected by these monogenic mutations listed in the latest update of *The Human*

Obesity Gene Map[17]. Thus it can be safely concluded that, however informative they are, the monogenic human obesities do not make a significant contribution to the global burden of disease. Despite much initial excitement, defects in the leptin gene have not turned out to be a wide-spread cause of obesity[17], and leptin so far shows very limited promise as a therapeutic agent for the general population[19].

Multigenic disorders

It has long been clear that overweight and obesity cluster in families; obesity is 2–8 times higher in the families of obese individuals than in the population at large and estimates of heritability range from 50–85% in twin studies down to 10–30% in adoption studies[10,20]. Quantitative trait analysis has found associations between obesity and genes on every human chromosome, but the associations are frequently refuted by subsequent investigations in different populations[17]. Likewise, candidate gene analysis, in which defects are searched for among genes which might reasonably be expected to lead to obesity, has tended to be disappointing. There has been a large number of negative findings and a tendency towards false positives for many of the findings which do initially suggest associations with various aspects of the obesity phenotype (*e.g.* BMI, fat distribution, maximal life-time body weight, age of onset of obesity, *etc*)[21].

There are several possible interpretations of this generally disappointing picture. The first has already been alluded to with reference to Figure 2, namely that obesity is a distal phenotype and arises after many years in which a range of environmental and social influences can displace the natural linkage between genotype and phenotype. The environmental factors may act independently of the genetic background (creating an entire shift in the population distribution), or there may be gene–environment interactions in which a person's susceptibility to a given environment is modified by their genes[11]. In the present context of early programming of the thrifty phenotype, it is interesting to note that the gene–environment interactions could also operate in the reverse direction since genetic expression is sensitive to diet at critical stages of development.

Although it is self-evident that gene–environment interactions must be important in determining obesity and other aspects of the metabolic syndrome related to the thrifty phenotype, they are very difficult to study in humans. Unfortunately, statistical constraints require the use of extremely large sample sizes even if the interactions are quite strong, and this seems likely to inhibit our future understanding of this important topic[22]. However, the study of gene–diet interactions has been successfully used in animal models in which selective breeding has been used to produce strains of mice that are highly susceptible or resistant to the obesity-inducing effects of a high-fat diet[23]. A similar genetic susceptibility to high-fat diets has been inferred in some human studies. For example, Heitman and colleagues demonstrated that only women with a family history of obesity appear to be susceptible to high-fat diets[24]. Another example in relation to the thrifty phenotype has recently emerged from the Isle of Ely study where Wareham and colleagues have demonstrated that a common mutation in the nuclear-receptor PPARγ alters fasting insulin levels, but that the effect is dependent on the P:S ratio of each subject's habitual diet (Wareham NJ, personal communication).

A further possible explanation for the disappointing progress in identifying common genetic causes of obesity is that their effects may be only significant when acting in concert with others – so-called gene–gene interactions[11]. Such interactions might simply be additive (where two genes acting in the same direction create a more noticeably distinct phenotype than either of them alone), or may be multiplicative (where one gene variant positively enhances the function of another). Recently, there have appeared several examples of claims of additive interactions emerging from candidate gene studies. For example, variants in the genes for uncoupling protein and the β_3-adrenoceptor have been reported to have an additive effect in causing morbid obesity[25]. However, caution must be exercised in interpreting such claims since the many possible combinations of gene x gene interactions are liable to throw up numerous false positive associations especially with the rather small sample sizes currently employed in such studies.

Insights into the mechanistic basis of obesity derived from genetic studies

The purpose of the above summary of genetic influences of obesity was to provide a perspective on the phenotypic influences described below and indicate how the two may interact. The genetic studies are currently driving progress into the understanding of the metabolic basis of obesity and in the course of just a few years have uncovered numerous new energy-regulatory pathways that lay hitherto unknown. A picture is emerging of bewildering complexity in which there is multiple overlap and redundancy between different neural networks with a wide range of feedback controls and tonic influences that have evolved to ensure, under most circumstances, an effective maintenance of energy balance. The complexity that is emerging humbles human efforts to summarise a mechanistic basis for obesity, and it is already proving necessary to develop 'in silico' models of metabolism in order to cope with the problem[26].

However, there are some key messages that can be extracted from this complexity and which may inform our future understanding of the metabolic basis of obesity. The first is that despite the exquisitely-evolved design characteristics of a control system that has served the human race for millennia, it is quite unable to cope with the profound environmental shift driven by the technological revolution at the end of the 20th century. In terms of our understanding of the possible effects of early-life programming, this implies that there is considerable plasticity in the extent to which genotype models phenotype. A second interesting observation is that all of the monogenic forms of extreme obesity in animals and man are mediated through defects in the appetite control side of the energy balance equation, rather than through the energy expenditure side. This may be because there is much greater scope to alter energy balance by altering intake than there is by altering expenditure[27], and is an observation that may be useful in moderating the past and persisting tendency to focus heavily on mechanisms mediated through defects in the regulation of expenditure.

Metabolic factors underlying susceptibility to obesity

In any given individual, the combination of their genetic background and their life-time exposures to diet and activity will create a metabolic setting which may be more or less susceptible to the obesogenic influences of the modern life-style. The possible routes through which this susceptibility might be mediated have commonly been clustered into a small group of possible explanatory theories. A very brief summary of some of the leading theories is provided below.

Slow metabolism

The theory that obesity resulted from an energy-sparing metabolic defect dominated research in this area for several decades. It had its origins in the misplaced belief that obese people do not overeat, and was given cogency by the unjustified extrapolation to man of the known defects in brown adipose tissue metabolism of the *ob/ob* mouse. Subsequent research has shown that obese people are characterised by a high energy expenditure and are hyperphagic[28–30]. In spite of many years' research throughout the world using techniques such as whole-body calorimetry and doubly-labelled water for measuring total energy expenditure, the mythical obese subject with a low metabolic rate has proved entirely elusive. Furthermore, many groups have now demonstrated that the apparently low energy intakes of obese people, which underpinned the search for putative metabolic defects, can be explained by profound under-reporting of energy intake by the obese[28,31,32].

Few people now subscribe to the low-metabolic-rate theory of obesity as a major aetiological route. However, Ravussin and colleagues demonstrated that a relatively low metabolic rate was a risk factor for weight gain in the Pima Indians[33], and in a recent review have concluded that it explains 12% of their susceptibility[34]. The discovery of the new uncoupling proteins (UCP2 and UCP3), which might be a source of energy-dissipating mechanisms in muscle and other tissues[35], has also renewed interest in this area despite the physiological evidence that obesity cannot be readily traced to a low energy expenditure[36]. Current evidence from genetic mapping suggests that neither UCP2 nor UCP3 are involved in the genetic transmission of obesity, though there is some evidence that polymorphisms in UCP1 may play a role[37]. The β_3-adrenergic receptor has also been the target of much interest because of its role as a specific receptor involved in stimulating thermogenesis in brown adipose tissue. Over 100 studies have explored associations between a β_3-adrenoceptor coding mutation (Trp64Arg) and obesity, but with very mixed results. About half claim an association and the other half fail to find any linkage[17,37].

Much of the current interest in the metabolic regulators of thermogenesis and energy expenditure is driven by the pharmaceutical industry which views the up-regulation of the β_3-adrenoceptor or of the UCPs as potential drug targets. The high level of research activity generated by this interest has a tendency to mislead the uninitiated into attributing to them a central role in the aetiology of obesity which probably would not be justified by a more objective assessment of the evidence. In the context of the early programming of a thrifty phenotype, it is unlikely that the transmission of any such effect is mediated through more than a very subtle effect on metabolic rate. Perhaps the strongest evidence for this comes from observations on Indians who can be assumed to have suffered a life-time of energy restriction and yet who fail to show any evidence of a low metabolic rate compared to well-nourished controls once appropriately adjusted for differences in body composition[38]. Our own research in The Gambia also reveals only subtle differences in metabolism between rural villagers who have been subjected to a life-time of under-nutrition and well-nourished Swiss controls once adjusted for differences in body weight[39].

Altered fuel selection

The energy balance equation (energy in – energy out = change in energy stores) can usefully be re-expressed in terms of each of the four energy-giving macronutrients (fat, carbohydrate, protein and alcohol)[40]. It can then be seen that the oxidation of fat must be equal to the sum of fat intake and any fat synthesis in order to avoid fat gain and ultimate obesity[41]. Any systematic displacement of the balance of fuel selection towards a low fat oxidation rate could gradually enhance fat deposition. The balance of fuel selection in an organism can be measured from the respiratory quotient (RQ) with a high RQ indicating high carbohydrate oxidation (and hence low fat oxidation).

The assessment of the characteristic RQ of an individual is difficult since it is highly variable over time as it responds to the short-term ebb and flow of energy balance and substrate availability between meals. The interpretation of data claiming to represent habitual RQ, therefore, requires caution. Nonetheless, a number of groups have shown a tendency towards an altered RQ in groups susceptible to obesity. A recent summary of the likely aetiological factors among the Pima Indians attributes 5% to the high RQ phenomenon[34]. Astrup and others have shown an altered fuel selection in post-obese patients, but the differences are small[42,43].

Differences in the muscle fibre-type profile have been postulated as a plausible physiological mechanism through which an altered fuel selection might be mediated. There is some evidence from exercise tests and muscle biopsies to support this suggestion[44], but others have failed to replicate this work[45]. On balance, the theory is attractive and could readily accommodate a long-term programming element if early-life nutrition caused a permanent anatomical resetting of fibre-type pattern. Phillips and colleagues have observed a number of metabolic differences in muscle according to size at birth confirming the possibility that this could be a route for programming and adjustment in fuel selection[46,47].

Adipose tissue hypercellularity

There is an extent to which adipose tissue depots regulate their own size. This accounts for the wide range of body shapes and the fact that fat distribution is more strongly inherited than absolute fat mass[48]. At the extreme end of the spectrum, the profoundly asymmetric fat distribution of patients suffering lipodystrophy underscores the importance of this level of autonomy of the fat stores.

Again this could provide a route for the long-term programming of a tendency towards obesity. Such a proposal was made several decades ago when the 'fat-cell number' theory postulated that early infant feeding (especially high-solute formula feeds) stimulated the creation of new adipocytes during a critical developmental window in infancy and that these were then permanently carried throughout life[49]. However, subsequent work has shown that fat cell numbers can increase beyond infancy, that adipocyte apoptosis can lead to a remodelling of fat cell numbers[50], and that there are very poor correlations between adipocity in infancy and in later life[49]. The constant fat-cell number theory is, therefore, no longer widely supported.

The refutation of the fat-cell number theory with respect to early-life programming does not invalidate the possibility that metabolic alterations which lead to an expansion of fat stores may be important in driving the positive energy balance which results in obesity. The reciprocal of this is also true; namely that any individual with very small numbers of adipocytes which show little tendency to hypertrophy will have nowhere to store excess lipid and may, therefore, have more powerful satiety signals and thus be resistant to weight gain. There is currently considerable interest in the factors regulating adipocyte hyperplasia and hence the control of fat depot size[50]. For instance, the terminal differentiation step in the conversion of pre-adipocytes into adipocytes is regulated by the nuclear-receptor PPARγ[51]. There are several natural ligands for this receptor which could induce fat cell division including some of the long-chain n-6 polyunsaturated fatty acids and their prostaglandin end products[52]. These could provide a link between diet composition and adipocity.

The possibility that glucocorticoids and stress may stimulate an excess deposition of intra-abdominal adipose tissue has been mooted for some years[53]. This may be of particular interest with respect to early programming of the thrifty phenotype in view of the evidence that maternal undernutrition may increase the exposure of the fetus to excess glucocorticoids[54] which in turn lead to a reduction in glucocorticoid receptors in the hippocampus and hence elevated levels of glucocorticoids in adult life[55]. There is some evidence that small size at birth is associated with a higher waist-hip ratio in adulthood[56].

Adipocytes also release a number of active peptides which may play a role in attempting to self-limit the expansion of the adipose tissue; including leptin, TNF-α, IL-6 and resistin[57,58]. It is conceivable that early programming effects might influence the tonic setting for the release of these compounds and hence alter the tendency towards adipocity. Evidence for the long-term programming of leptin has been published[59,60].

Altered 'set point'

Over the years, there has been much speculation and debate concerning the possibility that body weight is regulated according to a natural set point acting as a ponderostat or an adipostat by controlling the setting of regulatory feed-back loops linking appetite and energy expenditure. Experiments using hypothalamic lesions in rats strongly support such a concept by demonstrating that ventro-medial or lateral lesions will displace the natural growth trajectory and that the animals will then defend their growth along the new trajectory against both under- and over-feeding. There is strong evidence for some degree of set point control in humans, but it is clearly not an infallible system and an overly literal interpretation of the theory led it into disrepute for many years. During this period, Flatt developed the theory of a 'settling point' in which it was argued that body weight settled at a given level within any individual according to the balance of a number of metabolic factors; particularly the relationship between fat and carbohydrate oxidation[41].

The set point theory is making a strong come back (though in a more subtle guise) in view of the new molecular discoveries which have revealed the component elements necessary for the feedback control loops[14,16]. It would be easy to envisage ways in which early-life nutrition could adjust the position of the set-point and lead to a lifelong susceptibility or resistance to weight gain, but so far there is no concrete evidence.

Altered appetite control

As has been indicated, most of the monogenic examples of severe obesity are mediated through defects in appetite control, and simple calculations based on the natural variance of energy intake and energy expenditure confirm that there is much greater scope for displacing energy balance through changes in the energy intake side of the balance equation[27].

Our understanding of the factors regulating appetite and satiety is currently at an exciting cross-roads between the evidence gleaned from classic physiological experiments on appetite and the emerging insights based on newly discovered neural network pathways[61] and novel methods for imaging the activity of the brain[62]. The older evidence points to a range of physiological differences in satiety mechanisms between lean and obese people[63] especially in response to dietary fat[64], and to a variety of psychological syndromes associated with compulsive eating and addictive behaviours in relation to food in the obese[65]. New discoveries will ultimately explain these physiological and behavioural phenomena at a molecular level.

The question as to whether any of these 'satiety defects' could be pro-grammed by early-life events remains wide-open and has received little attention. In the short-term, there is evidence of a mixture of physio-logically and cognitively driven over-consumption following food deprivation[66] and this is probably responsible in part for weight rebound after restrictive dieting, but there is little evidence in support of longer-term influences. A single study reports the development of adult hyperphagia in rats subjected to fetal undernutrition[67], but such evidence would be very difficult to replicate in humans given the multiplicity of confounding events that occur between infancy and adulthood.

Behavioural and environmental factors

There is overwhelming evidence that the modern epidemic of obesity is caused by life-style changes over the past few decades that can be paraphrased[5,68] as 'gluttony and sloth'. Our analysis of the relative impact of gluttony and sloth on obesity rates in the UK suggests that it is the high levels of inactivity created by the technological revolution (and especially excess television viewing) which have been the dominant factor[68]. This is somewhat surprising conclusion in the light of comments made above about the greater scope of manipulating energy balance through changes in energy intake. Nonetheless, the evidence does suggest that at the **population** level it is inactivity which is creating the underlying susceptibility and at the **individual** level it is a failure to match appetite to these low levels of energy usage which is the key determinant of susceptibility.

Any putative effects of the early programming of a thrifty phenotype will be operating within these new environmental conditions and may show complex phenotype/environment interactions. The role of inactivity may emerge to be particularly important and will need to be factored into future research designs. For instance, it has been shown that adults who were small babies have alterations in muscle composition and metabolism[46,47]. It has also been shown that physical activity is a very powerful modulator of the cardiovascular metabolic syndrome[69]. This leaves plenty of scope for differences in activity patterns to have a major confounding effect on the emergence of the thrifty phenotype.

Excess adipose tissue as a cause of chronic disease

It may be useful to conclude with a reminder of the link between excess adipose tissue and the metabolic derangements associated with the thrifty phenotype, especially insulin resistance. It has been repeatedly shown that the development of obesity is the most important permissive factor which exposes the latent defects inherent in the thrifty phenotype. For many years, it was assumed that this was mediated through the release of high levels of fatty acids from adipose tissue, and that these caused insulin resistance through Randle Cycle competition with the utilisation of glucose, though this theory is now contested[70].

More recently, it has become apparent that adipose tissue is a highly active tissue releasing a broad range of bio-active signalling molecules

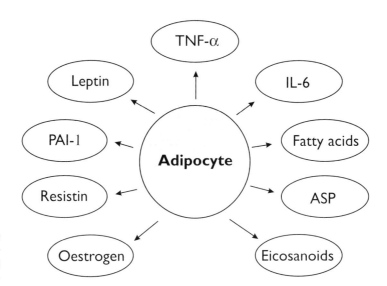

Fig 3 Adipose tissue as a source of bio-active signalling molecules.

which may influence insulin sensitivity (see Fig. 3)[57]. There has been great interest in the possibility that TNF-α may be the key link between adipocity and insulin resistance and there is much supporting evidence[71,72]. However, the very recent discovery of another new hormone, resistin, provides another candidate mediator for which there is provisional evidence of a very specific role in diabetes[58].

It is clear that future studies of the thrifty phenotype phenomenon and its link with obesity will need to explore modes of transmission involving these new molecular modulators of insulin action.

References

1   World Health Organization. *Obesity. Preventing and Managing the Global Epidemic*. Geneva: WHO, 1998
2   Phillips DI, Young JB. Birth weight, climate at birth and the risk of obesity in later life. *Int J Obes* 2000; **24**: 281–7
3   Byberg L, McKeigue PM, Zethelius B, Lithell HO. Birth weight and the insulin resistance syndrome: association of low birth weight with truncal obesity and raised plasminogen activator inhibitor-1 but not with abdominal obesity or plasma lipid disturbances. *Diabetologia* 2000; **43**: 54–60
4   Ravelli AC, Meulen JHvD, Osmond C, Barker DJ, Bleker OP. Obesity at the age of 50 y in men and women exposed to famine prenatally. *Am J Clin Nutr* 1999; **70**: 811–6
5   Prentice AM. Obesity – the inevitable penalty of civilisation? *Br Med Bull* 1997; **53**: 229–37
6   Neel JV. Diabetes mellitus: a 'thrifty' genotype rendered detrimental by 'progress'. *Am J Hum Genet* 1962; **14**: 353–62
7   Prentice AM. Fires of life: the struggles of an ancient metabolism in a modern world. *BNF Bull* 2001; **26**: 13–27
8   McGill HC, Mott GE, Lewis DS, McMahan CA, Jackson EM. Early determinants of adult metabolic regulation: effects of infant nutrition on adult lipid and lipoprotein metabolism. *Nutr Rev* 1996; **54**: S31–40

9   Hales CN, Barker DJP. Type 2 (non-insulin-dependent) diabetes mellitus: the thrifty phenotype hypothesis. *Diabetologia* 1992; **35**: 595–601

10   British Nutrition Foundation. *Obesity. Report of the BNF TaskForce*. Oxford: Blackwell, 1999

11   Barsh GS, Farooqi IS, O'Rahilly S. Genetics of body weight regulation. *Nature* 2000; **404**: 644–51

12   Various. Obesity (Nature Insight Series). *Nature* 2000; **404**: 631–77

13   Zhang Y, Proenca R, Maffei M, Barone M, Leopold L, Friedman JM. Positional cloning of the mouse gene and its human homologue. *Nature* 1994; **372**: 425–32

14   Friedman JM. Obesity in the new millenium. *Nature* 2000; **404**: 632–4

15   Tartaglia LA, Dempski M, Weng X et al. Identification and expression cloning of a leptin receptor, OB-R. *Cell* 1995; **83**: 1263–71

16   Friedman JM. Leptin, leptin receptors and control of body weight. *Eur J Med Res* 1997; **2**: 7–13

17   Chagnon YC, Perusse L, Weisnagel SJ, Rankinen T, Bouchard C. The human obesity gene map: the 1999 update. *Obes Res* 2000; **8**: 89–117 (also accessible electronically via http//www.obesite.chaire.ulaval.ca/genes.html)

18   Farooqi S, Jebb SA, Cook G et al. Recombinant leptin induces weight loss in human congenital leptin deficiency. *N Engl J Med* 1999; **341**: 879–84

19   Heymsfield SB, Greenberg AS, Fujioka K et al. Recombinant leptin for weight loss in obese and lean adults: a randomized controlled dose-escalation study. *JAMA* 1999; **282**: 1568–75

20   Maes HH, Neale MC, Eaves IJ. Genetic and environmental factors in relative body weight and human adiposity. *Behav Genet* 1997; **27**: 325–51

21   Clément J, Philip A, Jury C. Candidate gene approach of familial morbid obesity: linkage analysis of the glucocorticoid receptor gene. *Int J Obes* 1996; **20**: 507–12

22   Khoury MJ, Adams MJ, Flanders WD. An epidemiologic approach to ecogenetics. *Am J Hum Genet* 1988; **42**: 89–95

23   West DB, Waguespack J, McCollister S. Dietary obesity in the mouse: interaction of strain with diet composition. *Am J Physiol* 1995; **268**: R658–65

24   Heitmann BL, Lissner L, Sorensen TIA, Bengtsson C. Dietary fat intake and weight gain in women genetically predisposed for obesity. *Am J Clin Nutr* 1995; **61**: 1213–7

25   Clement K, Ruiz J, Cassard-Doulcier AM et al. Additive effect of A–>G (–3826) variant of the uncoupling protein gene and the Trp64Arg mutation of the beta 3-adrenergic receptor gene on weight gain in morbid obesity. *Int J Obes* 1996; **20**: 1062–6

26   Entelos. Entelos Obesity Physiolab:http//www.entelos.com/Products/obesitylab.html

27   Prentice AM, Jebb SA. Energy expenditure and regulation of human energy balance. In: Kopelman P. (ed) *Appetite, Obesity and Disorders of Over and Under-eating*. London: Royal College of Physicians, 1999; 13–21

28   Prentice AM, Black AE, Coward WA et al. High levels of energy expenditure in obese women. *BMJ* 1986; **292**: 983–7

29   Prentice AM, Black AE, Murgatroyd PR, Goldberg GR, Coward WA. Metabolism or appetite: questions of energy balance with particular reference to obesity. *J Hum Nutr Dietet* 1989; **2**: 95–104

30   Prentice AM, Black AE, Coward WA, Cole TJ. Energy expenditure in affluent societies: an analysis of 319 doubly labelled water measurements. *Eur J Clin Nutr* 1996; **50**: 93–7

31   Lichtman SW, Pisarska K, Berman E et al. Discrepancy between self-reported and actual caloric intake and exercise in obese subjects. *N Engl J Med* 1993; **327**: 1893–8

32   Schoeller DA. How accurate is self-reported dietary energy intake? *Nutr Rev* 1990; **48**: 373–9

33   Ravussin E, Lillioja S, Knowler W et al. Reduced rate of energy expenditure as a risk factor for body weight gain. *N Engl J Med* 1988; **318**: 467–72

34   Ravussin E, Bogardus C. Energy balance and weight regulation: genetics versus environment. *Br J Nutr* 2000; **83**: S17–20

35   Lowell BB, Spiegelman BM. Towards a molecular understanding of adaptive thermogenesis. *Nature* 2000; **404**: 652–9

36   Schrauwen P, Walder K, Ravussin E. Human uncoupling proteins and obesity. *Obes Res* 1999; 7: 97–105

37 Arner P. Obesity – a genetic disease of adipose tissue? *Br J Nutr* 2000; **83 (Suppl 1)**: S9–16
38 Shetty PS. Chronic undernutrition and metabolic adaptation. *Proc Nutr Soc* 1993; **52**: 267–84
39 Minghelli G, Schutz Y, Charbonnier A, Whitehead R, Jequier E. Twenty-four hour energy expenditure and basal metabolic rate measured in a whole-body calorimeter in Gambian men. *Am J Clin Nutr* 1990; **51**: 563–70
40 Prentice AM. Are all calories equal? In: Cottrell R. (ed) *Weight Control: The Current Perspective*. London: Chapman & Hall, 1995; 8–33
41 Flatt J-P. Importance of nutrient balance in body weight regulation. Diabetes 1988; **4**: 571–81
42 Astrup A, Buemann B, Toubro S, Raben A. Defects in substrate oxidation involved in the predisposition to obesity. *Proc Nutr Soc* 1996; **55**: 817–28
43 Astrup A, Buemann B, Christiansen NJ, Toubro S. Failure to increase lipid oxidation in response to increasing dietary fat content in formerly obese women. *Am J Physiol* 1994; **266**: E592–9
44 Wade A, Marbut MM, Round JM. Muscle fibre type and aetiology of obesity. *Lancet* 1990; **335**: 805–8
45 Geerling BJ, Alles MS, Murgatroyd PR, Goldberg GR, Harding M, Prentice AM. Fatness in relation to substrate oxidation during exercise. *Int J Obes* 1994; **18**: 453–9
46 Thompson CH, Sanderson AL, Sandeman D et al. Fetal growth and insulin resistance in adult life: role of skeletal muscle morphology. *Clin Sci* 1997; **92**: 291–6
47 Phillips DI, Caddy S, Ilic V et al. Intramuscular triglyceride and muscle insulin sensitivity: evidence for a relationship in non-diabetic subjects. *Metabolism* 1996; **45**: 947–50
48 Bouchard C. Genetic determinants of regional fat distribution. *Hum Reprod* 1997; **12 (Suppl 1)**: 1–5
49 Poskitt EME. Do fat babies stay fat? *BMJ* 1977; **i**: 7–9
50 Prins JB, O'Rahilly S. Regulation of adipose cell number in man. *Clin Sci* 1997; **92**: 3–11
51 Vidal-Puig A, Jimenez-Linan M, Lowell BB et al. Regulation of PPAR-gamma gene expression by nutrition and obesity in rodents. *J Clin Invest* 1996; **97**: 2553–61
52 Ailhaud G, Grimaldi P, Negrel R. Cellular and molecular aspects of adipose tissue development. *Annu Rev Nutr* 1992; **12**: 207–33
53 Bjorntorp P. The regulation of adipose tissue distribution in humans. *Int J Obes* 1996; **20**: 291–302
54 Langley SC, Phillips G, Benediktsson R et al. Maternal dietary protein restriction, placental glucocorticoid metabolism and the programming of hypertension. *Placenta* 1996; **17**: 169–72
55 Phillips DI, Fall CHD, Seckl JR et al. Elevated plasma cortisol concentrations: an explanation for the relationship between low birthweight and adult cardiovascular risk factors. *J Clin Endocrinol Metab* 1998; **83**: 757–60
56 Fall CH, Osmond C, Barker DJ et al. Fetal and infant growth and cardiovascular risk factors in women. *BMJ* 1995; **310**: 428–32
57 Mohamed-Ali V, Pinkney J, Coppack S. Adipose tissue as an endocrine and paracrine organ. *Int J Obes* 1998; **22**: 1145–58
58 Steppan CM, Bailey ST, Bhat S et al. The hormone resistin links obesity to diabetes. *Nature* 2001; **409**: 307–12
59 Lissner L, Karlsson C, Lindroos AK et al. Birth weight, adulthood BMI, and subsequent weight gain in relation to leptin levels in Swedish women. *Obes Res* 1999; **7**: 150–4
60 Phillips DI, Fall CH, Cooper C, Norman RJ, Robinson JS, Owens PC. Size at birth and plasma leptin concentrations in adult life. *Int J Obes* 1999; **23**: 1025–9
61 Schwartz MW, Woods SC, Porte D, Seeley RJ, Baskin DG. Central nervous system control of food intake. *Nature* 2000; **404**: 661–71
62 Gautier JF, Chen K, Salbe AD et al. differential brain responses to satiation in obese and lean men. *Diabetes* 2000; **49**: 838–46
63 Rolls B, Kim-Harris S, Fischmann M, Foltin R. Satiety after preloads with different amounts of fat and carbohydrate: implications for obesity. *Am J Clin Nutr* 1994; **60**: 476–87
64 Blundell J, Macdiarmid J. Fat as a risk factor for overconsumption: satiation, satiety and patterns of eating. *J Am Dietet Assoc* 1997; **97**: S63–9
65 Jebb SA, Prentice AM. Is obesity an eating disorder? *Proc Nutr Soc* 1995; **B**: 721–8

66   Keys AJ, Brozek J, Henschel O, Michelson O, Taylor HL. *The Biology of Human Starvation*. Minnesota: University of Minnesota Press, 1950

67   Vickers MH, Breier BH, Cutfield WS, Hofman PL, Gluckman PD. Fetal origins of hyperphagia, obesity, and hypertension and postnatal amplification by hypercaloric nutrition. *Am J Physiol* 2000; **279**: E83–7

68   Prentice AM, Jebb SA. Obesity in Britain: gluttony or sloth? *BMJ* 1995; **311**: 437–9

69   Wareham NJ, Hennings SJ, Byrne CD, Hales CN, Prentice AM, Day NE. A quantitative analysis of the relationship between habitual energy expenditure, fitness and the metabolic cardiovascular syndrome. *Br J Nutr* 1998; **80**: 235–41

70   Kelley DE, Mandarino LJ. Fuel selection in human skeletal muscle in insulin resistance: a re-examination. *Diabetes* 2000; **49**: 677–83

71   Hotamisligil G, Spiegelman B. Tumour necrosis factor α: a key component of the obesity-diabetes link. *Diabetes* 1994; **43**: 1271–8

72   Hotamisligil G. The role of TNF alpha and TNF receptors in obesity and insulin resistance. *J Intern Med* 1999; **245**: 621–5

The malnourished baby and infant

David J P Barker

MRC Environmental Epidemiology Unit, Southampton General Hospital, Southampton, UK

The growth of a baby is constrained by the nutrients and oxygen it receives from the mother. A mother's ability to nourish her baby is established during her own fetal life and by her nutritional experiences in childhood and adolescence, which determine her body size, composition and metabolism. Mother's diet in pregnancy has little effect on the baby's size at birth, but nevertheless programmes the baby. The fetus adapts to undernutrition by changing its metabolism, altering its production of hormones and the sensitivity of tissues to them, redistributing its blood flow, and slowing its growth rate. In some circumstances, the placenta may enlarge. Adaptations to undernutrition that occur during development permanently alter the structure and function of the body.

Fetal nutrition

The supply of nutrients to the fetus is the major influence that regulates its growth. It depends on the mother's body composition and size, her nutrient stores, what she eats during pregnancy, transport of nutrients to the placenta and transfer across it. This long and vulnerable series of steps is known as the fetal supply line. The fetus becomes undernourished when its demand for nutrients exceeds its supply. Either the supply may be low, for example when the mother is thin or starving or when the placenta fails, or demand may be high because the fetus is growing rapidly.

Early in development, before implantation, the embryo comprises two groups of cells, the inner cell mass which becomes the fetus and the outer cell mass which becomes the placenta. Experiments in animals indicate that the allocation of cells between the two masses is influenced by nutrition and by hormones[1,2]. In experimental animals, maternal undernutrition at the time of conception leads to fewer cells in the inner cell mass, which is associated with reduced birth weight and postnatal growth, altered organ/body weight ratios and the development of hypertension[3]. Better periconceptual nutrition is thought to raise the fetal growth trajectory[4] which is established in early gestation when the fetus' absolute requirement for nutrients is small. A more rapid growth trajectory leads to an increased demand for nutrients in late gestation,

Correspondence to:
Prof. David J P Barker,
MRC Environmental
Epidemiology Unit,
Southampton General
Hospital, Tremona Road,
Southampton
SO16 6YD, UK

when requirements are relatively large and when the progressive reduction in the ratio of placental to fetal size reduces placental reserve capacity[5]. The fetus' ability to sustain growth during a period of under-nutrition depends on its previous growth rate, more rapidly growing fetuses with a high demand for nutrients being less able to sustain growth[6,7]. Males grow more rapidly than females and are, therefore, less able to withstand undernutrition.

Because the fetus' requirements for nutrients are small in early gestation, it is often assumed that undernutrition will not influence growth until late gestation, when substrate supply becomes inadequate to meet increasing fetal demand for tissue building blocks. This is not, however, the case. When, for example, female pigs are fed low protein diets from the time of mating the weight and length of their fetuses are already reduced at mid-gestation[8]. This indicates that fetal under-nutrition can affect fetal growth through mechanisms other than lack of substrate supply to growing tissues.

Fetal adaptations to undernutrition

In common with other living things, the human fetus is able to adapt to undernutrition. Its responses include metabolic changes, redistribution of blood flow and changes in the production of fetal and placental hormones which control growth[9]. They are shown in Figure 1. Its immediate metabolic response to undernutrition is catabolism: it consumes its own substrates to provide energy[8]. More prolonged undernutrition leads to a slowing in growth rate. This enhances the fetus' ability to survive by reducing the use of substrates and lowering the metabolic rate. Slowing of growth in late gestation leads to disproportion in organ size since organs and tissues that are growing rapidly at the time are affected the most. For example, undernutrition in late gestation may lead to reduced growth of the kidney which is developing rapidly at that time. Reduced replication of kidney cells may permanently reduce cell numbers, because after birth there seems to be no capacity for renal cell division to 'catch-up'[10,11].

Animal studies show that a variety of different patterns of fetal growth result in similar birth size. For example, a fetus that grows slowly through-out gestation may have the same size at birth as a fetus whose growth was arrested for a period and then 'caught up'. Different patterns of fetal growth will have different effects on the relative size of different organs at birth, even though overall body size may be the same. This emphasises the severe limitation of birth weight as a measure of fetal growth.

While slowing its rate of growth, the fetus may protect tissues that are important for immediate survival, the brain especially. One way in which the brain can be protected is by redistribution of blood flow to

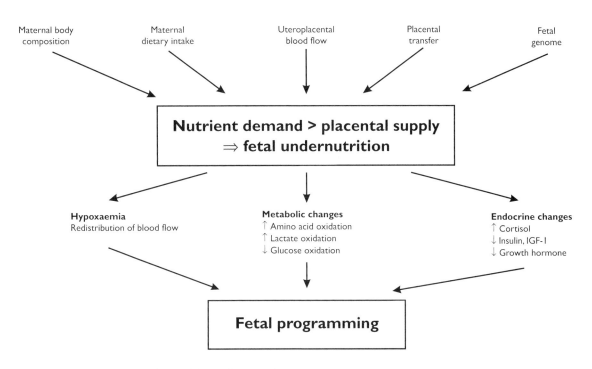

Fig. 1 Fetal adaptations to undernutrition: a framework.

favour it[12,13]. This adaptation is known to occur in many mammals but in humans it may have exaggerated costs for other tissues, notably the liver and other abdominal viscera, because of the large size of the brain.

It is becoming increasingly clear that nutrition has profound effects on fetal hormones, and on the hormonal and metabolic interactions between the fetus, placenta and mother on whose co-ordination fetal growth depends[8]. Fetal insulin and the insulin-like growth factors (IGFs) are thought to have a central role in the regulation of growth and respond rapidly to changes in fetal nutrition[14]. If a mother decreases her food intake, fetal insulin, IGF-1 and glucose concentrations fall, possibly through the effect of decreased maternal growth hormone and IGF This leads to reduced transfer of amino acids and glucose from mother to fetus, and ultimately to reduced rates of fetal growth[15]. In late gestation and after birth, the fetus' growth hormone and IGF axis take over, from insulin, a central role in driving linear growth. Whereas undernutrition leads to a fall in the concentrations of hormones that control fetal growth, it leads to a rise in cortisol whose main effect is on cell differentiation[9].

The differing effects of undernutrition at different stages of gestation may be summarised as follows[16].

Early pregnancy

As has been described already, the concentrations of nutrients in the earliest stages of pregnancy influence growth of the embryo. Animal studies have shown that birth size can be profoundly changed by a brief period of *in vitro* culture before implantation. Sub-optimal nutrition before implantation retards growth and development, the one-cell embryo being particularly sensitive. The early embryo is selective in its use of nutrients and respires pyruvate, lactate, and amino acids such as glutamine rather than glucose[4]. Before implantation it switches to a glucose-based metabolism, and low glucose concentrations retard its growth and development[17]. Paradoxically, perhaps, high glucose concentrations, which accompany maternal diabetes, also delay embryonic growth. This effect contrasts with the accelerated growth associated with high glucose concentrations in late pregnancy.

Mid-pregnancy

The placenta grows faster than the fetus in mid-pregnancy and nutrient deficiency may, therefore, affect fetal growth by changing the interaction between the fetus and the placenta. Whereas maternal undernutrition restricts growth of fetus and placenta, mild undernutrition may lead to increased placental, but not fetal, size[18]. This placental overgrowth may be an adaptation to sustain nutrient supply from the mother. Localised placental hypertrophy can also be induced experimentally in sheep by reducing the number of implantation sites. Owens and Robinson[19] have shown that the compensatory growth at the remaining sites occurs before there is noticeable retardation of fetal growth, and may be a sensitive, early response to reduced nutrient supply.

During undernutrition, fetal growth may be sacrificed to maintain placental function. In animals oxygen, glucose and amino acids may be redistributed, so that the placenta reduces its consumption of oxygen and glucose while maintaining a large output of lactate to the fetus[20]. The lactate is partly derived from amino acids of fetal origin, and the fetus may waste and be thin at birth[20]. There is evidence for similar metabolic changes in growth retarded human fetuses, in whom wasting has been observed by ultrasonography[21-23].

Late pregnancy

In late gestation, undernutrition results in immediate slowing of fetal growth. Acute undernutrition causes prompt slowing of fetal growth associated with fetal catabolism[6], but fetal growth rapidly resumes when nutrition is restored. In contrast, prolonged undernutrition may irreversibly slow the rate of fetal growth in lambs and lead to reduced length at birth[24]. The basis of this irreversibility is uncertain, but it is reflected in the clinical observation that children with intra-uterine growth retardation who show postnatal growth failure are those with evidence of more prolonged intra-uterine growth retardation[25].

Mother's height and smoking

Mother's height is related to birth weight: short women have small babies[26]. Teleologically, this form of constraint can be viewed as a way of ensuring that the fetus cannot outgrow the size of the mother's pelvis and birth canal. Mother's skeletal size is not, however, related to the long-term changes in the physiology and metabolism of the fetus which are described in this issue[16,27]. Similarly, while mother's cigarette smoking is associated with reduced birth weight, it does not appear to be associated with long-term changes in glucose/insulin metabolism. Consistent with this, neither mother's height, smoking habits or age are related to cord blood insulin concentrations whereas mother's dietary intakes of carbohydrate and protein are strongly associated with cord blood concentrations of insulin and its precursors[28]. This chapter, therefore, focuses on other influences that determine delivery of nutrients to the fetus.

Genes and fetal growth

Although the growth of a fetus is influenced by its genes, studies in humans and animals suggest that it is usually limited by the nutrients and oxygen it receives[29,30]. The mother seems to exert a stronger effect on fetal growth than the father. Among half siblings, related only through one parent, those with the same mother have similar birth weights, the correlation coefficient being 0.58. The birth weights of half siblings with the same father are, however, dissimilar, the correlation coefficient being only 0.1[31]. Other studies of relatives have shown that first cousins related through the mother tend to have similar birth weights whereas paternal first cousins do not[32]. Penrose analysed the birth weights of relatives and concluded that 62% of the variation between individuals was the result of the intra-uterine environment, 20% was the result of maternal genes and 18% of fetal genes[33]. A study of babies born after ovum donation showed that while their birth weights were strongly related to the weight of the recipient mother (Fig. 2), they were unrelated

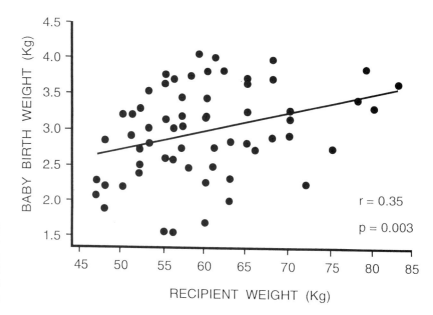

Fig. 2 Birth weight of babies born after ovum donation according to weight of the recipient mother.

to the weight of the woman who donated the egg[34]. Studies in domestic animals also suggest that birth size is essentially controlled by the mother rather than the genetic inheritance from both parents[26,35-37]. In Walton and Hammond's well known experiments, in which Shetland and Shire horses were crossed, the foals were smaller at birth when the Shetland pony was the mother than when the Shire horse was the mother[38]. As the genetic composition of the two crosses was similar, this implied that the Shetland mother had constrained the growth of the fetus.

Genes and fetal adaptations

Little is known about the genes which underlie the fetal cardiovascular, metabolic and hormonal adaptations to undernutrition. Genes which allow the fetus to adapt successfully to undernutrition are likely to be favoured by natural selection even though they may lead to disease and premature death in post-reproductive life. The fundamental role of genetic information is to enable the cell and organism to maintain homeostasis in the face of environmental changes, that is to maintain the intracellular concentrations necessary for survival, while the supply of these from external sources fluctuate. Common genetic variation results in different individuals in a population having differing ability to maintain homeostasis under different environmental challenges. In response to poor nutrient availability *in utero*, some fetuses will fail to make appropriate homeostatic responses and will die; some will make responses that will allow growth to continue at the same rate; others will make homeostatic responses that will ensure survival but the growth rates of some tissues and systems will slow. This last group will be at risk of coronary heart disease and other disorders in adult life.

Maternal–fetal conflict

Haig and others have suggested that the relation between mother and fetus can usefully be viewed as genetic conflict[39,40]. The effects of natural selection on genes expressed in fetuses may be opposed by the effects of natural selection on genes expressed in mothers. Fetal genes will be selected to increase the transfer of nutrients to the fetus so that it grows larger. Maternal genes will be selected to limit transfer to the fetus to protect the mother, and to ensure her survival and that of her children, born and unborn. What is best for the fetus need not be best for its mother, or so it seems.

The theory of parent–child conflict proposes that children are selected to demand more resources from parents than parents are selected to give. Three sets of genes have different interests: the mother's genes, the fetus' genes derived from the mother, and the fetus' genes derived from the father. If the genes of the fetus make excessive demands on the mother, it will prejudice the mother's ability to pass her genes on to other offspring. It is argued that genes derived from the father have been selected to take more resources from the mother's tissues than the genes derived from the mother[41]. The conflict between the maternal and paternal genomes over the nutritional demands that the fetus imposes on its mother may explain why genes derived from one parent can 'imprint', or override, the expression of those derived from the other[42]. An example of 'genomic imprinting' is that of the genes for insulin-like growth factor II. In the mouse, only those derived from the father are expressed[43,44].

An interesting example of the conflict of interests between mother and baby, though it is not genetic conflict, comes from the breeding habits of southern elephant seals[45]. They come ashore to breed on the island of South Georgia and nourish their pups only from the reserves of fat and protein stored in their bodies on arrival at the beaches. The proportion of the food reserves made available to the pups may be critical to both mother and child. Mothers that expend a large proportion on their pups may compromise their survival to the next breeding season or reduce their subsequent reproductive output. On the other hand, pups that are small and thin have reduced chances of survival to breeding age. The production of small pups by smaller mothers may be a compromise between the future reproductive success of the mother and the survival of the pup. Male pups are heavier at birth than females and the smallest elephant seal mothers only give birth to females, which suggests that they abort male pups. This may be an advantage if they are unable to raise a male pup to a viable size without jeopardising their own survival and reproductive success.

When animals breed before they are mature maternal–fetal conflict may be enhanced. James has suggested that whereas the hormonal responses to pregnancy in adult women seem geared to optimising the flow of nutrients to the fetus, the opposite seems to occur when adolescent girls are pregnant[46]. Paradoxically, feeding young pregnant adolescent lambs leads to a selective channelling of nutrients to the mother who thrives at the expense of the fetus.

Maternal nutrition and body size at birth

Fetal nutrition must be distinguished from maternal nutrition. Experience in famine shows that even extreme restrictions in mother's food intake during pregnancy have only modest effects on birth weight. From this it cannot be concluded that fetal growth is not regulated by its nutrient supply. Rather it suggests that maternal nutrient intakes during pregnancy have relatively small effects on birth size, which may depend more on mother's nutritional state before pregnancy – on the turnover of her protein and fatty acid stores in her muscle and fat. Birth weight is a crude measure of fetal growth: babies of the same weight may, for example, be short and fat or long and thin, and may be markedly different in organ size and structure, physiology and metabolism. The next sections describe what is known about the effects of maternal body composition and diet on birth size, body proportions at birth, and placental growth.

Mother's body size before pregnancy

A mother's body size before pregnancy is the most important determinant of the size of her baby. The variation in body form around the world is changing rapidly, which must have profound consequences for fetal growth. Whereas in Western countries many women are slim by choice, around the world most women with low body weight in relation to their height have been chronically undernourished since childhood. Women who have low body weight before pregnancy have small babies[47–50]. Chronic undernutrition also influences birth weight through its effect on maternal stature, independent of body weight[26,51]. It may also be associated with deficiencies in specific nutrients which influence fetal growth, including vitamins A, C, and D, folate, iron and zinc[52].

Among chronically undernourished mothers, high weight gain during pregnancy partly offsets the effects of low weight before pregnancy, although the babies' weights still tend to remain below average[53,54]. The mother stores fat in the first half of pregnancy and mobilises it in the second under the influence of placental growth hormone and other hormones. In this way she spares glucose for the fetus by switching to fat as her primary energy source. Observations on weight gain in obese women point to the importance of pre-pregnant weight in determining birth weight. Those who gain little weight during pregnancy, or even lose weight, still have babies of average or above average weight[53–57].

Differences in the proportions of fat in different parts of the body are known to be linked to differences in metabolism and hormonal profile. Deposition of fat on the abdomen, for example, is associated with resistance to insulin and an altered balance of sex hormones[58], and fat at different sites on the body makes varying amounts of oestrogen. The effects that the hormonal and metabolic variations which are linked to body fat distribution have on the fetus are largely unknown.

Weight gain and diet during pregnancy

In Europe, mothers gain around 12 kg (26 lb) in weight during pregnancy. The maternal component of this averages 7.7 kg (17 lb) and comprises increases in fat, extracellular fluid, uterine and breast tissue. Maternal fat stores of around 3 kg (7 lb) are mostly laid down during the first half of pregnancy and provide an energy store for the fetus in late gestation. The extracellular fluid volume is increased by 3 l. Half of this increase is due to expansion of the plasma volume which, together with a fall in the peripheral resistance and increase in heart rate, leads to an increase in cardiac output. The cardiac output increases by 40% during the first trimester. Plasma volume increases more if the fetus is large and the mother's cardiovascular adaptations, which determine the perfusion of the placenta, are important determinants of fetal nutrition. We know little about the effects of the mother's body composition and nutrition before pregnancy on these adaptations[59].

In Western countries, except in extreme circumstances, maternal undernutrition during pregnancy, reflected in low maternal weight gain, leads to only modest reductions in birth weight[60–63]. Indeed, the weak relationship between maternal weight gain in pregnancy and birth size has contributed to the myth that, in affluent populations, nutrition has little effect on fetal growth[64]. This myth arises from failure to understand the importance of maternal body composition, itself determined by nutrition, failure to distinguish fetal from maternal nutrition, and the use of crude indicators of fetal growth such as birth weight.

During the past 50 years, numerous studies have examined whether the quality of the diet eaten by a pregnant woman influences the birth weight of the baby. The results have been various and contradictory[65]. The relationship between calorie intake in pregnancy and birth weight, found in observational studies and trials, is of varying size and generally less than had been expected[66]. In one of the best known studies in Aberdeen, Scotland, the diets of primagravid women were recorded by weighed food intakes and food diaries during the seventh month of pregnancy[67]. Calorie intake was associated with birth weight in that women who consumed less than 1800 calories per day had babies who weighed 240 g (0.5 lb) less than those of mothers who ate 3000 and more calories, but this is a small effect.

The Dutch hunger winter lasted for 5 months and daily calorie intakes fell below 1000. Babies exposed to the famine during the first half of gestation, who were born after the famine was lifted, had normal birth weight. Those exposed during the second half of gestation had lower birth weight, being 327 g (0.7 lb) lighter than babies born before the famine[68,69]. The effect of the famine in Wuppertal, Germany, during 1945–1946 was less. Calorie intake was reduced to around 2400 a day and birth weight was reduced by around 185 g (0.4 lb)[70]. The exceptionally severe famine in Leningrad (now St Petersburg) during 1941–1943 led to a 530 g (1.2 lb) fall in mean birth weight[71]. The German blockade of Leningrad between September 1941 and January 1944 prevented supplies from reaching the city for 900 days. During the siege, approximately 1 million Leningrad citizens died from a total population of 2.4 million. Most of these deaths occurred during the 'hunger winter' of November 1941 to February 1942 when the siege was in full force and the average daily ration was about 300 calories, composed almost entirely of carbohydrate. Nearly 50% of all term infants exposed to famine during the second half of gestation weighed less than 2.5 kg (5.5 lb).

In some trials, supplementation of the mother's diet has led to an increase in mean birth weight, though generally of small size. One trial of protein-calorie supplementation, among poorly nourished mothers in New York City, produced a fall in mean birth weight[72]. This unexpected result led to a re-analysis of all reported supplementation trials[73]. Supplements with a low percentage of calories as protein were found to have increased birth weight whereas supplements with a high protein density reduced birth weight.

A number of studies support the idea that the inconsistency in the results of different trials could be the result of differing effects in women whose nutritional status differed before pregnancy. Underweight women with high calorie intakes during pregnancy have babies of similar size to those of overweight women with low calorie intakes. A trial among

Asian women living in England suggested that the babies of women whose triceps skinfold thickness did not increase in mid-pregnancy benefited most from protein and energy supplementation[74]. In The Gambia, energy supplementation increased birth weight only during the wet season, a time when food is scarce and women work hard planting crops[75]. In the New York study, only the babies of mothers who smoked cigarettes benefited[72]; whether this reflected the different diets of smokers and non-smokers is not known.

Maternal nutrition and body proportions at birth

Animal studies show that fetal undernutrition at different times in gestation may lead to new-borns with different overall body size or with similar body size but marked differences in the proportional size of different organs. In sheep, for example, undernutrition in late pregnancy increases the weight of the heart without altering body size. Chronic nutritional deprivation sustained from early pregnancy is associated with proportionate growth failure in head size, length, and weight[5,36]. Undernutrition in mid or late gestation is associated with disproportionate growth, reflected in thinness or shortness at birth. This is, of course, an over-simplification. Though thinness at birth may result from failure of nutrient supply in late pregnancy, this failure may originate from influences affecting placental development in early gestation[76]. The guinea pig fetus becomes thin only if the mother is continuously undernourished from early or mid pregnancy to term, while it will become short if the mother is undernourished in early or mid pregnancy only.

There is limited information about the maternal influences that determine different body proportions at birth. Figure 3 shows that the babies of mothers who had low birth weight tend to be thin irrespective of the mother's current body size[77]. In that particular study, maternal stature had no additional effect, though Kramer has found that taller mothers tend to have longer, thinner babies[78]. The father's birth weight did not influence ponderal index but taller fathers have longer, thinner babies[77]. Low dairy protein intake in late pregnancy is also associated with thinness at birth and Dutch babies exposed to wartime famine in the last trimester were thin[69,79]. Other studies have shown that reduced protein intake in pregnancy is associated with shortness at birth[80].

An important difference between fetal growth in non-industrialised countries and that in Western countries is that proportionate growth retardation is common in the non-industrialised countries whereas disproportionate, or 'asymmetrical', growth retardation prevails in Western countries[36]. Babies with proportionate growth retardation may be more prone to neurodevelopmental impairment, whereas those with

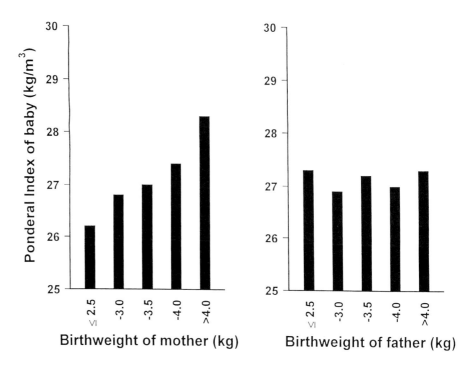

Fig. 3 Ponderal index at birth of 492 term babies according to the birth weight of their mothers and fathers.

disproportionate growth retardation may be more at risk of perinatal death[81-83].

Maternal nutrition and the placenta

Placental size and the ratio of placental weight to birth weight have been found to be associated with type 2 diabetes and impaired glucose tolerance. Among 7086 men and women born in Helsinki, those who developed type 2 diabetes tended to have had low placental weight as well as low birth weight[84]. In contrast, glucose tolerance tests performed on 226 men and women born in Preston, UK, showed that those with impaired glucose tolerance or type 2 diabetes had an increased ratio of placental weight to birth weight[85].

Maternal undernutrition has variable effects on placental growth. In general, it has little effect in early and late gestation: in mid-gestation its effects vary. Some animal studies have shown that maternal under-nutrition in mid-pregnancy reduces placental weight[86,87]. Others have shown increased placental weight (in sheep), or an increase in the ratio of placental to fetal weight (in guinea-pigs)[18,88,89]. The findings in sheep are not readily reproducible and McCrabb suggested that this might be the result of different maternal nutritional reserves before conception[89]. Subsequently, Robinson and colleagues in Adelaide showed that good nutrition around the time of conception followed by a restricted diet in mid-pregnancy, stimulated placental growth in sheep, whereas mid-pregnancy undernutrition in an already poorly nourished ewe restricted placental growth[90]. These observations on the effect of a changing plane of nutrition during pregnancy are consistent with empirical practices in sheep farming, whereby ewes are moved from rich pasture to poor pasture after mating. If they are then returned to rich pasture in later pregnancy, the lambs are heavier than those whose mothers were on rich pasture throughout. These surprising observations inevitably raise questions about the effects of nausea and anorexia in human pregnancy.

In humans, there is some evidence that high food intakes in mid-pregnancy may also suppress placental growth. A study of the diets of an unselected group of pregnant women suggested that high intakes of carbohydrates in mid-pregnancy, especially simple carbohydrates such as are found in soft drinks, suppressed placental growth[91]. This was especially marked if high carbohydrate intake in mid-pregnancy was followed by low dairy protein intake in late pregnancy. Differential effects of carbohydrates on placental size were also found in a recent trial. In this instance, however, 'aboriginal' carbohydrates, which are associated with a lower blood sugar after ingestion led to reduced placental and fetal size[92].

In contrast to the apparent suppressive effect of carbohydrate, Beischer showed that anaemia during pregnancy was associated with increased placental size[93]. In a study of 8684 pregnant women in Oxford, those whose haemoglobin concentrations fell to lower values during pregnancy had larger placentas[94]. Subsequent studies showed that among women with low haemoglobin, placental volume was already increased at 18 weeks of pregnancy[95]. Furthermore, Wheeler and colleagues showed that maternal haemoglobin concentrations between 9–11 weeks of pregnancy were inversely related to the maternal serum concentrations of chorionic gonadotrophin and placental lactogen – hormones synthesised by the placenta[96]. The associations between maternal haemoglobin and placental size and function are not explained by the effects of haemodilution. They may reflect the effects of a reduced oxygen content in maternal blood. Hypoxia may stimulate blood vessel formation in the growing placenta by increasing the expression of angiogenic growth factors such as vascular endothelial growth factor.

The mild hypoxaemia associated with life at high altitude is also associated with an increase in the ratio of placental to fetal weight[97,98]. Clapp has shown that if mothers exercise vigorously in early pregnancy the volume of the placenta in mid-pregnancy is increased[99]. Cigarette smoking suppresses both placental and fetal growth but suppression of the placenta is less and the ratio of placental to fetal weight at birth is therefore increased[97]. These effects may also be mediated by hypoxia, though other influences must also affect the ratio of placental to fetal weight, which is raised if the mother has a high body mass[100].

Further evidence that the placental enlargement may be an adaptive response to lack of oxygen or nutrients comes from a study of babies that were unusually small (below the 10th centile) for their gestational age[101]. Their ratio of placental to birth weight was higher than that of babies whose size was appropriate to their gestational age.

Intergenerational constraints on fetal growth

In addition to the effects of mother's body composition and diet on birth weight, mothers' birth weights are related to those of their children and even their children's children[102–107]. Women who were small for gestational age at birth are at twice the risk of having a small for gestational age baby and their babies are more likely to die in the perinatal period[107,108]. Women who had low birth weight also tend to have thin babies. The father's birth weight has no effect on ponderal index[77], though it influences placental weight. These observations have led to the conclusion that mothers constrain fetal growth and that the degree of constraint they exert is set when they themselves are *in utero*[109]. 'Maternal constraint' is thought to reflect the limited capacity of the mother to deliver nutrients to her fetus[110]. Sisters, who experience a common level of constraint *in utero*, exert a similar level of constraint on their own fetuses. Although low birth weight is a feature of the families of mothers who have growth retarded babies, it is not a feature of the families of the fathers. Studies of babies who are unusually large at birth have shown, however, that large birth weight is common in the families of both parents. One interpretation of this is that the father influences the fetal growth trajectory only when maternal constraint is relaxed[109]. We do not know the mechanisms by which a mother's poor fetal growth impairs the fetal growth of her offspring, but one possibility is that a reduced uterine vasculature is laid down *in utero* and this impairs placentation in the next generation.

Fifty years ago, Mussey wrote[111]: 'it must be borne in mind that the diet of a given generation may affect the offspring several generations hence'. This has been demonstrated experimentally in animals. Stewart under-nourished a colony of rats with a protein deficient diet over 12 generations. When he re-fed them with a normal diet, it took 3 generations before fetal growth and development were restored to normal[112]. Similarly, the adverse effects of exercise in pregnancy on fetal growth in rats are evident in the second generation[113]. It follows that in humans who move from poorly nourished to well nourished communities, Indian migrants to Europe for example, it will take more than one generation before fetal growth increases to the level of the host country[114].

The realisation that a mother's physiological capacity to nourish her fetus was established when she herself was *in utero* is not new. Mellanby wrote[115]: 'it is certain that the significance of correct nutrition in child-bearing does not begin in pregnancy itself or even in the adult female before pregnancy. It looms large as soon as a female child is born and indeed in its intra-uterine life'. Hence the fetus adapts its rate of growth, and the life-long structure and function of its body, not only to its mother, but to the environment its grandmother provided for its mother. Sensitivity to more than one generation allows the fetus to adapt to the level of nutrition which has prevailed over many years rather than only to that at the time of its conception. This may be important in places where there is periodic famine.

Long-term effects of maternal nutrition on glucose-insulin metabolism

In the Dutch famine study, it was people born to mothers who had low body weight who had the highest plasma glucose concentrations 2 h after a standard glucose load[116]. A study of middle-aged men and women in Scotland suggested that an association between low maternal body mass index and insulin resistance in the offspring might underlie this observation[117]. This observation has been confirmed in a study of men and women in Beijing, China (Table 1), and found to apply to body mass index in both early and late pregnancy[118]. An interpretation of this is that the association between maternal body mass and insulin resistance is initiated in early pregnancy. Table 2 shows similar findings in a group of older men and women in Finland[119]. In these people, the associations between low maternal body mass index and offspring's plasma glucose, insulin and pro-insulin concentrations were independent of the offspring's body size at birth and during childhood. The particular aspect of maternal metabolism that is associated with low body mass index and leads to insulin resistance is not known, but low protein turnover is one possibility. The relationship between mother's diet in pregnancy and the glucose-insulin metabolism of the offspring in

Table 1 2-h plasma glucose and insulin concentrations in Chinese men and women aged 45 years according to mother's body mass index (BMI) at 15 weeks of pregnancy

Variable	Mother's BMI					
	≤19.2	−20.5	−22.3	> 22.3	All	*P* value
No. of subjects	56	57	57	56	226	
2-h glucose (mmol/l)	7.4	7.0	7.1	5.6	6.7	0.008
2-h insulin (pmol/l)	399	299	252	181	273	0.02

Table 2 Plasma glucose and insulin concentrations in Finnish men and women aged 69 years, according to maternal body mass index in late pregnancy

	Maternal body mass index (kg/m^2)						
	≤24	–25.5	–27	–29	> 29	All	P value
No. of subjects	87	87	86	90	86	436	
Fasting glucose (nmol/l)*	5.5	5.5	5.7	5.5	5.4	5.5	0.44
2-h glucose (nmol/l)*	8.0	7.8	8.6	7.1	7.2	7.7	0.007
Fasting insulin (pmol/l)*	78	71	68	60	63	68	0.01
2-h insulin (pmol/l)*	582	551	519	474	412	504	<0.001
Fasting pro-insulin (pmol/l)	3.5	3.5	3.0	2.8	2.6	3.0	0.001
Fasting 32-33 split pro-insulin (pmol/l)	8.6	8.8	7.8	7.8	7.2	8.0	0.08

Values are adjusted for age and sex only.
*Values are geometric means.

middle age was examined in the Scottish study. The offspring of mothers with high intakes of fat and protein in late pregnancy had a reduced plasma insulin increment between fasting and 30 min[117]. This was independent of the association between high maternal body mass and low insulin increment, an association which studies of gestational diabetes suggest may be mediated by raised maternal plasma glucose concentrations (*see* Fall, this issue).

References

1   Kleeman DO, Walker SK, Seamark RF. Enhanced fetal growth in sheep administered progesterone during the first three days of pregnancy. *J Reprod Fertil* 1994; **102**: 411–7
2   Walker SK, Hartwich KM, Seamark RF. The production of unusually large offspring following embryo manipulation: concepts and challenges. *Theriogenology* 1996; **45**: 111–20
3   Kwong WY, Wild A, Roberts P, Willis AC, Fleming TP. Maternal undernutrition during the preimplantation period of rat development causes blastocyst abnormalities and programming of postnatal hypertension. *Development* 2000; **127**: 4195–202
4   Leese HJ. Heyner S, Wiley L. (eds) *Early Embryo Development and Paracrine Relationships*. New York: Alan R. Liss, 1990; 67–78
5   Woods DL, Bruton MN. (eds) *Alternative Life-History Styles of Animals*. Dordrecht: Kluwer, 1989; 459–64
6   Harding J, Liu L, Evans P, Oliver M, Gluckman P. Intrauterine feeding of the growth retarded fetus: can we help? *Early Hum Dev* 1992; **29**: 193–7
7   Widdowson EM, McCance RA. The effect of finite periods of undernutrition at different ages on the composition and subsequent development of the rat. *Proc R Soc Lond B Biol Sci* 1963; **158**: 329–42
8   Harding JE, Johnston BM. Nutrition and fetal growth. *Reprod Fertil Dev* 1995; **7**: 539–47
9   Fowden AL. Endocrine regulation of fetal growth. *Reprod Fertil Dev* 1995; **7**: 351–63
10 Widdowson EM, Elliott K, Knight J. (eds) *Size at Birth. Ciba Symposium 27*. Amsterdam: Elsevier, 1974; 65–82
11 Hinchliffe SA, Lynch MRJ, Sargent PH, Howard CV, Van Velzen D. The effect of intrauterine growth retardation on the development of renal nephrons. *Br J Obstet Gynaecol* 1992; **99**: 296–301

12 Campbell AGM, Dawes GS, Fishman AP, Hyman AI. Regional redistribution of blood flow in the mature fetal lamb. *Circ Res* 1967; **21**: 229–35

13 Rudolph AM. The fetal circulation and its response to stress. *J Dev Physiol* 1984; **6**: 11–9

14 Fowden AL. The role of insulin in prenatal growth. *J Dev Physiol* 1989; **12**: 173–82

15 Oliver MH, Harding JE, Breier BH, Evans PC, Gluckman PD. Glucose but not a mixed amino acid infusion regulates plasma insulin-like growth factor-1 concentrations in fetal sheep. *Pediatr Res* 1993; **34**: 62–5

16 Barker DJP, Gluckman PD, Godfrey KM, Harding JE, Owens JA, Robinson JS. Fetal nutrition and cardiovascular disease in adult life. *Lancet* 1993; **341**: 938–41

17 Gott AL, Hardy K, Winston RML, Leese HJ. Non-invasive measurement of pyruvate and glucose uptake and lactate production by single human preimplantation embryos. *Hum Reprod* 1990; **5**: 104–8

18 McCrabb GJ, Egan AR, Hosking BJ. Maternal undernutrition during mid-pregnancy in sheep. Placental size and its relationship to calcium transfer during late pregnancy. *Br J Nutr* 1991; **65**: 157–68

19 Owens JA, Robinson JS. Cockburn F. (eds) *Fetal and Neonatal Growth*. Chichester: Wiley, 1988; 49–77

20 Owens JA, Falconer J, Robinson JS. Effect of restriction of placental growth on fetal and utero-placental metabolism. *J Dev Physiol* 1987; **9**: 225–38

21 Divon MY, Chamberlain PF, Sipos L, Manning FA, Platt LD. Identification of the small for gestational age fetus with the use of gestational age-independent indices of fetal growth. *Am J Obstet Gynecol* 1986; **155**: 1197–201

22 Soothill PW, Nicolaides KH, Campbell S. Prenatal asphyxia, hyperlacticaemia, hypoglycaemia and erythroblastosis in growth retarded fetus. *BMJ* 1987; **294**: 1051–3

23 Cetin I, Corbetta C, Sereni LP *et al*. Umbilical amino acid concentrations in normal and growth-retarded fetuses sampled *in utero* by cordocentesis. *Am J Obstet Gynecol* 1990; **162**: 253–61

24 Mellor DJ, Murray L. Effects on the rate of increase in fetal girth of refeeding ewes after short periods of severe undernutrition during late pregnancy. *Res Vet Sci* 1982; **32**: 377–82

25 Fancourt R, Campbell S, Harvey D, Norman AP. Follow-up study of small-for-dates babies. *BMJ* 1976; **i**: 1435–7

26 Cawley RH, McKeown T, Record RG. Parental stature and birth weight. *Ann Hum Genet* 1954; **6**: 448–56

27 Forsen T, Eriksson JG, Tuomilehto J, Teramo K, Osmond C, Barker DJP. Mother's weight in pregnancy and coronary heart disease in a cohort of Finnish men: follow up study. *BMJ* 1997; **315**: 837–40

28 Godfrey KM, Robinson S, Hales CN, Barker DJP, Osmond C, Taylor KP. Nutrition in pregnancy and the concentrations of proinsulin, 32-33 split proinsulin, insulin, and C-peptide in cord plasma. *Diabet Med* 1996; **13**: 868–73

29 McCance RA, Widdowson EM. The determinants of growth and form. *Proc R Soc Lond B Biol Sci* 1974; **185**: 1–17

30 Gluckman PD, Breier BH, Oliver M, Harding J, Bassett N. Fetal growth in late gestation – a constrained pattern of growth. *Acta Paediatr Scand Suppl* 1990; **367**: 105–10

31 Morton NE. The inheritance of human birth weight. *Ann Hum Genet* 1955; **20**: 123–34

32 Robson EB. Birth weight in cousins. *Ann Hum Genet* 1955; **19**: 262–8

33 Penrose LS. Some recent trends in human genetics. *Caryologia* 1954; **6 (Suppl)**: 521–30

34 Brooks AA, Johnson MR, Steer PJ, Pawson ME, Abdalla HI. Birth weight: nature or nurture? *Early Hum Dev* 1995; **42**: 29–35

35 Lush JL, Hetzer HO, Culbertson CC. Factors affecting birth weights of swine. *Genetics* 1934; **19**: 329–43

36 Kline J, Stein Z, Susser M. *Conception to Birth – Epidemiology of Prenatal Development*. New York: Oxford University Press; 1989

37 Roberts DF, Falkner F, Tanner JM. (eds) *Human Growth, vol 3, Methodology: Ecological, Genetic and Nutritional Effects on Growth*. New York: Plenum, 1986

38 Walton A, Hammond J. The maternal effects on growth and conformation in Shire horse–Shetland pony crosses. *Proc R Soc Lond B Biol Sci* 1938; **125**: 311–35

39 Trivers RL. Parent-offspring conflict. *Am Zool* 1974; **14**: 249–64

40   Moore T, Haig D. Genomic imprinting in mammalian development: a parental tug of war. *Trends Genet* 1991; **7**: 45–9

41   Haig D, Graham C. Genomic imprinting and the strange case of the insulin-like growth factor II receptor. *Cell* 1991; **64**: 1045–6

42   Lyle R. Gametic imprinting in development and disease. *J Endocrinol* 1997; **155**: 1–12

43   Hall JG. Genomic imprinting: review and relevance to human diseases. *Am J Hum Genet* 1990; **46**: 857–73

44   De Chiara TM, Robertson EJ, Efstratiadis A. Parental imprinting of the mouse insulin-like growth factor II gene. *Cell* 1991; **64**: 849–59

45   Fedak MA, Arnbom T, Boyd IL. The relation between the size of southern elephant seal mothers, the growth of their pups, and the use of maternal energy, fat, and protein during lactation. *Physiol Zool* 1996; **69**: 887–911

46   James WPT. Long-term fetal programming of body composition and longevity. *Nutr Rev* 1997; **55**: S41–3

47   Tompkins WT, Wiehl DG, Mitchell RM. The underweight patient as an increased obstetric hazard. *Am J Obstet Gynecol* 1955; **69**: 114–23

48   Love EJ, Kinch RAH. Factors influencing the birth weight in normal pregnancy. *Am J Obstet Gynecol* 1965; **91**: 342–9

49   Edwards LE, Alton IR, Barrada MI, Hakanson EY. Pregnancy in the underweight woman. Course, outcome, and growth patterns of the infant. *Am J Obstet Gynecol* 1979; **135**: 297–302

50   Naeye RL, Blanc W, Paul C. Effects of maternal nutrition on the human fetus. *Pediatrics* 1973; **52**: 494–503

51   Baird D. The influence of social and economic factors on stillbirths and neonatal deaths. *J Obstet Gynaecol Br Empire* 1945; **52**: 339–66

52   Backstrand JR, Allen LH. Boulton J, Laron Z, Rey J. (eds) *Long-Term Consequences of Early Feeding*. Philadelphia, PA: Lippincott-Raven, 1995

53   Eastman NJ, Jackson E. Weight relationships in pregnancy. I. The bearing of maternal weight gain and pre-pregnancy weight on birth weight in full term pregnancies. *Obstet Gynecol Surv* 1968; **23**: 1003–25

54   Rosso P. Nutrition and maternal-fetal exchange. *Am J Clin Nutr* 1981; **34**: 744–55

55   Simpson JW, Lawless RW, Mitchell AC. Responsibility of the obstetrician to the fetus. *Obstet Gynecol* 1975; **45**: 481–7

56   Edwards LE, Dickes WF, Alton IR, Hakanson EY. Pregnancy in the massively obese: course, outcome, and obesity prognosis of the infant. *Am J Obstet Gynecol* 1978; **131**: 479–83

57   Abrams BF, Laros RK. Pre-pregnancy weight, weight gain, and birth weight. *Am J Obstet Gynecol* 1986; **154**: 503–9

58   Bjorntorp P. Adipose tissue distribution and function. *Int J Obes* 1991; **15**: 67–81

59   Capeless EL, Clapp JF. Cardiovascular changes in early phase of pregnancy. *Am J Obstet Gynecol* 1989; **161**: 1449–53

60   Susser M. Maternal weight gain, infant birthweight and diet: causal sequences. *Am J Clin Nutr* 1991; **53**: 1384–96

61   Niswander K, Jackson EC. Physical characteristics of the gravida and their association with birth weight and perinatal death. *Am J Obstet Gynecol* 1974; **119**: 306–13

62   Gormican A, Valentine J, Satter E. Relationships of maternal weight gain, pre-pregnancy weight, and infant birthweight. *J Am Diet Assoc* 1980; **77**: 662–7

63   Hytten FE, Chamberlain G. *Clinical Physiology in Obstetrics*. Oxford: Blackwell Scientific, 1980

64   Editorial: Maternal nutrition and low birth-weight. *Lancet* 1975; **ii**: 445

65   Rosso P. *Nutrition and Metabolism in Pregnancy – Mother and Fetus*. New York: Oxford University Press, 1990

66   Lechtig A, Klein RE. Dobbing J. (eds) *Maternal Nutrition in Pregnancy – Eating for Two?* London: Academic Press, 1981; 131–74

67   Thomson AM. Diet in pregnancy. 3. Diet in relation to the course and outcome of pregnancy. *Br J Nutr* 1959; **13**: 509–25

68   Smith CA. The effect of wartime starvation in Holland upon pregnancy and its product. *Am J Obstet Gynecol* 1947; **53**: 599–608

69 Stein Z, Susser M, Saenger G *et al*. *Famine and Human Development: The Dutch Hunger Winter of 1944/45*. New York: Oxford University Press, 1975
70 Dean RFA. *Studies of Undernutrition. Wuppertal 1946–9*. London: HMSO, 1951; 346–78
71 Antonov AN. Children born during the siege of Leningrad in 1942. *J Pediatr* 1947; **30**: 250–9
72 Rush D, Stein Z, Susser M. A randomized controlled trial of prenatal nutritional supplementation in New York City. *Pediatrics* 1980; **65**: 683–97
73 Rush D, Sharp F, Fraser RB, Milner RDG. (eds) *Fetal Growth*. London: Royal College of Obstetricians and Gynaecologists, 1989; 203–33
74 Viegas OAC, Scott PH, Cole TJ, Eaton P, Needham PG, Wharton BA. Dietary protein energy supplementation of pregnant Asian mothers at Sorrento, Birmingham. II: selective during third trimester only. *BMJ* 1982; **285**: 592–5
75 Prentice AM, Whitehead RG, Watkinson M, Lamb WH, Cole TJ. Prenatal dietary supplementation of African women and birth-weight. *Lancet* 1983; **ii**: 489–92
76 Robinson JS, Owens JA, de Barro T *et al*. Maternal nutrition and fetal growth. In: Ward RHT, Smith SK, Donnai D. (eds) *Early Fetal Growth and Development*. London: Royal College of Obstetricians and Gynaecologists, 1994; 317–34
77 Godfrey KM, Barker DJP, Robinson S, Osmond C. Maternal birthweight and diet in pregnancy in relation to the infant's thinness at birth. *Br J Obstet Gynaecol* 1997; **104**: 663–7
78 Kramer MS, Olivier M, McLean FH, Dougherty GE, Willis DM, Usher RH. Determinants of fetal growth and body proportionality. *Pediatrics* 1990; **86**: 18–26
79 Stein Z, Susser M. The Dutch Famine 1944–45 and the reproductive process. I. Effects on six indices at birth. *Pediatr Res* 1975; **9**: 70–6
80 Burke BS, Harding VV, Stuart HC. Nutrition studies during pregnancy IV. Relation of protein content of mother's diet during pregnancy to birth length, birth weight, and condition of infant at birth. *J Pediatr* 1948; **32**: 506–15
81 Walther FJ, Ramaekers LHJ. Neonatal morbidity of SGA infants in relation to their nutritional status at birth. *Acta Paediatr Scand* 1982; **71**: 437–40
82 Villar J, Smeriglio V, Martorell R, Brown CH, Klein RE. Heterogeneous growth and mental development of intrauterine growth-retarded infants during the first 3 years of life. *Pediatrics* 1984; **74**: 783–91
83 Haas JD, Balcazar H, Caulfield L. Variation in early neonatal mortality for different types of fetal growth retardation. *Am J Phys Anthropol* 1987; **73**: 467–73
84 Forsen T, Eriksson J, Tuomilehto J, Reunanen A, Osmond C, Barker D. The fetal and childhood growth of persons who develop type 2 diabetes. *Ann Intern Med* 2000; **133**: 176–82
85 Phipps K, Barker DJP, Hales CN, Fall CHD, Osmond C, Clark PMS. Fetal growth and impaired glucose tolerance in men and women. *Diabetologia* 1993; **36**: 225–8
86 Everitt GC. Maternal undernutrition and retarded foetal development in Merino sheep. *Nature* 1964; **201**: 1341–2
87 Wallace AM. The growth of lambs before and after birth in relation to the level of nutrition. *J Agric Sci* 1984; **38**: 243–302
88 Faichney GJ, White GA. Effects of maternal nutritional status on fetal and placental growth and on fetal urea synthesis in sheep. *Aust J Biol Sci* 1987; **40**: 365–77
89 McCrabb GJ, Egan AR, Hosking BJ. Maternal undernutrition during mid-pregnancy in sheep; variable effects on placental growth. *J Agric Sci* 1992; **118**: 127–32
90 DeBarro 1M, Owens J, Earl CR *et al*. Nutrition during early/mid pregnancy interacts with mating weight to affect placental weight in sheep [Abstract]. *Australian Society for Reproductive Biology*, Adelaide 1992
91 Godfrey K, Robinson S, Barker DJP, Osmond C, Cox V. Maternal nutrition in early and late pregnancy in relation to placental and fetal growth. *BMJ* 1996; **312**: 410–4
92 Clapp J, Ridzon S, Lopez B *et al*. Diet, exercise, and feto-placental growth [Abstract]. *J Soc Gynecol Invest* 1996; **3** (**Suppl 2**): 273A
93 Beischer NA, Sivasamboo R, Vohra S, Silpisornkosal S, Reid S. Placental hypertrophy in severe pregnancy anaemia. *J Obstet Gynaecol Br Commonwealth* 1970; **77**: 398–409
94 Godfrey KM, Redman CWG, Barker DJP, Osmond C. The effect of maternal anaemia and iron deficiency on the ratio of fetal weight to placental weight. *Br J Obstet Gynaecol* 1991; **98**: 886–91

95 Howe D, Wheeler T. Maternal iron stores and placental growth [Abstract]. *J Physiol* 1993; **467**: 290

96 Wheeler T, Sollero C, Alderman S, Landen J, Anthony F, Osmond C. Relation between maternal haemoglobin and placental hormone concentrations in early pregnancy. *Lancet* 1994; **343**: 511–3

97 Meyer MB, Reed DM, Stanley FJ. (eds) *The Epidemiology of Prematurity*. Baltimore, MD: Urban and Schwarzenberg, 1977; 81–104

98 Mayhew TM, Jackson MR, Haas JD. Oxygen diffusive conductances of human placentae from term pregnancies at low and high altitudes. *Placenta* 1990; **11**: 493–503

99 Clapp JF, Rizk KH. Effect of recreational exercise on midtrimester placental growth. *Am J Obstet Gynecol* 1992; **167**: 1518–21

100 Williams LA, Evans SF, Newnham JP. Factors influencing the relative growths of the fetus and the placenta [Abstract]. *Proceedings of the Australian Perinatal Society* 1996; A46

101 Lao TT, Wong WM. Placental ratio and intrauterine growth retardation. *Br J Obstet Gynaecol* 1996; **103**: 924–6

102 Hackman E, Emanuel I, van Belle G, Daling J. Maternal birth weight and subsequent pregnancy outcome. *JAMA* 1983; **250**: 2016–9

103 Klebanoff MA, Graubard B, Kessel SS, Berendes HW. Low birth weight across generations. *JAMA* 1984; **252**: 2423–7

104 Carr-Hill R, Campbell DM, Hall MH, Meredith A. Is birth weight determined genetically? *BMJ* 1987; **295**: 687–9

105 Alberman E, Emanuel I, Filakti H, Evans SJW. The contrasting effects of parental birthweight and gestational age on the birthweight of offspring. *Paediatr Perinat Epidemiol* 1992; **6**: 134–44

106 Emanuel I, Filakti H, Alberman E, Evans SJW. Intergenerational studies of human birthweight from the 1958 birth cohort. I. Evidence for a multigenerational effect. *Br J Obstet Gynaecol* 1992; **99**: 67–74

107 Klebanoff MA, Meirik O, Berendes HW. Second-generation consequences of small-for-dates birth. *Pediatrics* 1989; **84**: 343–7

108 Skjaerven R, Wilcox AJ, Oyen N, Magnus P. Mothers' birth weight and survival of their offspring: population based study. *BMJ* 1997; **314**: 1376–80

109 Ounsted M, Scott A, Ounsted C. Transmission through the female line of a mechanism constraining human fetal growth. *Ann Hum Biol* 1986; **13**: 143–51

110 Gluckman P, Harding J, Hernandez M, Argente J. (eds) *Human Growth: Basic and Clinical Aspects*. Amsterdam: Elsevier, 1992; 253–9

111 Mussey RD. Nutrition and human reproduction: an historical review. *Am J Obstet Gynecol* 1949; **57**: 1037–48

112 Stewart RJC, Sheppard H, Preece R, Waterlow JC. The effect of rehabilitation at different stages of development of rats marginally malnourished for ten to twelve generations. *Br J Nutr* 1980; **43**: 403–12

113 Pinto ML, Shetty PS. Influence of exercise-induced maternal stress on fetal outcome in Wistar rats: inter-generational effects. *Br J Nutr* 1995; **73**: 645–53

114 Dhawan S. Birth weights of infants of first generation Asian women in Britain compared with second generation Asian women. *BMJ* 1995; **311**: 86–8

115 Mellanby E. Nutrition and child-bearing. *Lancet* 1933; **2**: 1131–7

116 Ravelli ACJ, van der Meulen JHP, Michels RPJ *et al*. Glucose tolerance in adults after prenatal exposure to famine. *Lancet* 1998; **351**: 173–7

117 Shiell AW, Campbell DM, Hall MH, Barker DJP. Diet in late pregnancy and glucose-insulin metabolism of the offspring 40 years later. *Br J Obstet Gynaecol* 2000; **107**: 890–5

118 Mi J, Law CM, Zhang KL, Osmond C, Stein CE, Barker DJP. Effects of infant birthweight and maternal body mass index in pregnancy on components of the insulin resistance syndrome in China. *Ann Intern Med* 2000; **132**: 253–60

119 Eriksson J, Forsen T, Jaddoe VWV, Osmond C, Barker DJP. The effects of childhood growth and maternal body size on insulin resistance in elderly men and women. *Diabelologica 2002*; In press

The role of genetic susceptibility in the association of low birth weight with type 2 diabetes

Timothy M Frayling and **Andrew T Hattersley**

Department of Diabetes and Vascular Medicine, School of Postgraduate Medicine and Health Sciences, University of Exeter, Exeter, UK

We suggest that altered fetal growth and type 2 diabetes may be two phenotypes of the same genotype – in other words the 'thrifty phenotype' is the result of a 'thrifty genotype'. Supporting this there is strong evidence that paternal factors and, therefore, genes influence fetal growth and that these paternal genes affecting fetal growth may also alter diabetes risk. Further study is needed to determine whether common gene variants can explain the association between reduced birth weight and increased risk of type 2 diabetes. If the genetic hypothesis is true, common diabetes genes are likely to have subtle effects on insulin secretion and/or action and, therefore, subtle effects on fetal growth. Large cohorts of infants and their parents will be required – probably in the region of thousands rather than hundreds – to identify gene variants that may explain the association between reduced birth weight and increased risk of type 2 diabetes. All previously described associations between birth weight and type 2 diabetes have required many hundreds of subjects and it is likely that the geneticists and the 'programmists' are trying to identify very subtle physiological effects.

*Correspondence to:
Dr Tim M Frayling,
Department of Diabetes
and Vascular Medicine,
School of Postgraduate
Medicine and Health
Sciences, University of
Exeter, Barrack Road,
Exeter EX2 5AX, UK
T.M.Frayling@exeter.ac.uk*

There is no doubt that low birth weight is associated with adult disorders characterised by insulin resistance such as type 2 diabetes, hypertension, dyslipidaemia and coronary heart disease[1–3]. However, the mechanism of this established association is still uncertain and controversial. For the past decade, research has principally focused on the role of the intra-uterine environment. It has been proposed that undernutrition *in utero* results in a permanent re-programming of the fetal metabolism[1]. Genetic factors are not part of this thrifty phenotype hypothesis, but there is a significant body of evidence suggesting that they are important both as determinants of birth weight and adult diseases like type 2 diabetes. We have proposed a hypothesis that low birth weight and type 2 diabetes are two phenotypes of the same insulin resistant genotype (Fig. 1)[4]. In this chapter, we put forward some of the

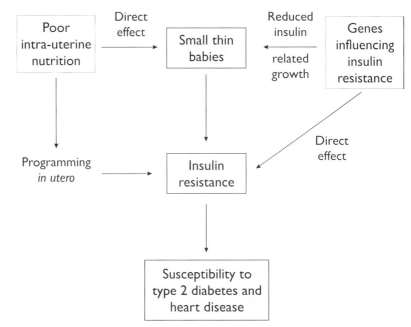

Fig. 1 Genes or environment? The two explanations for the association between low birth size and type 2 diabetes, insulin resistance and ischaemic heart disease (adapted from Hattersley & Tooke[4]).

arguments for genetic explanations as an alternative to the thrifty phenotype hypothesis. We would accept that these two mechanisms are not exclusive and it is likely that the adult phenotype of diseases like type 2 diabetes is a reflection of the genotype **and** the intra-uterine **and** the post-natal environment with different factors having different predominance in different individuals.

Low birth weight and type 2 diabetes: genes can explain the association

Genetic variation is a potential explanation of the association between birth weight and adult disorders such as type 2 diabetes. In the 'fetal insulin hypothesis'[4], we proposed that gene variants that result in differences in insulin resistance or secretion within the normal population may also affect birth weight and size through effects on insulin-mediated fetal growth. The crucial components of this proposal are that: (i) genetic susceptibility is important for both birth weight and diabetes; and (ii) genes that reduce insulin secretion or increase insulin resistance will predispose to small babies as well as to diabetes. Finally, it will be important to define the relative role of these genes compared to the impact of the intra-uterine environment. This is not just a sterile intellectual debate, but will give fundamental insights into the aetiology of adult disease and the most appropriate prevention strategies.

The predisposition to type 2 diabetes is influenced by genes

Type 2 diabetes results from the interaction of genetic susceptibility and a permissive environment. The prevalence of type 2 diabetes and the 'metabolic syndrome' is rapidly increasing due to environmental and behavioural changes such as the increasingly sedentary life-style and high-fat, high-refined carbohydrate diet. This does not exclude a role for genes as the risk of type 2 diabetes for a given individual is likely to reflect their genetic predisposition as well as their activity and obesity (factors which in turn may be partially genetic (reviewed by Vogler *et al*[5]). There is a large amount of evidence to suggest an individual's susceptibility to diabetes is, at least in part, genetically determined. Type 2 diabetes and insulin resistance clusters in families with siblings of patients having a 3–4-fold increased risk of developing the disease compared to members of the general population[6–8]. Monozygotic twins have higher concordance rates than dizygotic twins[9]. Populations at high risk of diabetes remain at high risk when they migrate to countries associated with a low prevalence of type 2 diabetes[10]. Some of these observations can be put down to shared environment as well as, or instead of, shared genes. Stronger evidence comes from population admixture studies[11,12]. For example, in the high prevalence native-American Pima Indian population, the risk of diabetes is altered by the degree of genetic admixture from low prevalence populations such as Caucasians despite apparently identical environments[12]. Furthermore, recent successes in the mapping of type 2 diabetes genes demonstrates that genes are important in determining who develops type 2 diabetes. Variants in the *Calpain 10* gene[13] and the regulatory 'VNTR' region of the insulin gene[14] are linked with type 2 diabetes risk.

Birth weight is influenced by genetic factors – the importance of paternal as well as maternal factors

There is considerable evidence that genetic factors are important in the determination of fetal birth weight. There is greater variation in birth size between non-identical twins than identical twins[15] There are also clear paternal effects on fetal growth *in utero*. Mothers have two ways of influencing the growth and health of their unborn offspring – their DNA and the intra-uterine environment. Fathers can influence the unborn offspring solely through their DNA. There are, therefore, numerous strong correlations between maternal factors and fetal growth parameters (*see* Barker, this issue). There is much evidence, however, that indicates fathers also influence the growth and development of their unborn child. In a study of 538 infants born in Southampton, birth weight, length and placental weight were all highly significantly correlated with the father's own birth weight and height[16]. In a simultaneous regression analysis, birth weight showed the strongest independent association with paternal birth weight and height[16].

Studies of agricultural animals, where body size and composition are important economic variables, also indicate that genes as well as maternal environment affect birth weight. Studies of cattle demonstrate that breed of sire influences birth weight as well as other important growth traits[17,18]. There is evidence of a genetic effect on birth weight and growth from the classic study of Shetland pony/Shire horse crosses performed in the 1930s. These studies demonstrated that foals closely resembled in size the mare's size at birth, perhaps unsurprisingly given the vast differences between the two breeds. However, foals born to Shire mares and Shetland stallions tended to be smaller at birth and were significantly smaller than pure bred Shires after 4 months' growth (see Barker, this issue, for further discussion)[19].

The central role of insulin in both fetal growth and carbohydrate regulation: a possible common pathway for the influence of genes

What are the potential mechanisms whereby genes could influence fetal growth and also the development of diabetes? Insulin secretion and insulin action are excellent candidate pathways as insulin plays a key role both in carbohydrate regulation and also in fetal growth (see Fowden & Hill, this issue). Impaired insulin action and secretion are the two features common to type 2 diabetes[20]. Fetal insulin secretion is one of the key determinants of fetal growth acting mainly in the third trimester when the weight of the fetus increases markedly. The clearest clinical example of this is the macrosomic children born to mothers with diabetes in pregnancy. Pedersen proposed that this macrosomia did not result from a direct increase in the transfer of nutrients, but was mediated indirectly by increased fetal insulin secretion in response to fetal sensing of maternal hyperglycaemia[21]. In pregnant mothers with diabetes or glucose intolerance, the maintenance of maternal euglycaemia, particularly in the third trimester, reduces the risk of macrosomia[22]. The evidence for the important role of insulin comes not only from diabetic pregnancies. In normal pregnancies, there is a direct correlation between the maternal blood glucose levels in the third trimester of pregnancy and the birth weight of the child[23–26].

Fetal insulin mediated growth may not only reflect maternal glycaemia (altering the stimulus to fetal insulin secretion) but also fetal genetic factors which regulate the fetus' insulin secretion and the sensitivity of

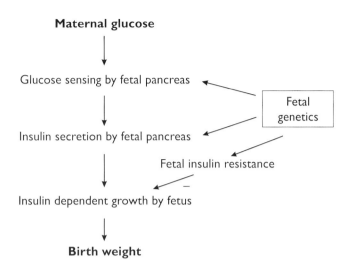

Fig. 2 The fetal insulin hypothesis. A simplified diagram of how fetal genetics may alter birth weight through insulin mediated growth (adapted from Hattersley & Tooke[4]).

fetal tissues to the effects of insulin. As the fetus produces insulin in response to the maternal glucose level, then a genetic defect in either the sensing of the maternal glucose by the fetal pancreas, or insulin secretion by the fetal pancreas, or the action of the insulin on the insulin-dependent tissues, would all result in reduced fetal growth (Fig. 2). There is now support for this 'fetal insulin hypothesis' which is outlined below.

Evidence for the role of genes in birth weight and type 2 diabetes: single gene disorders of insulin secretion and action alter fetal growth

Observations of fetal development in single gene disorders that alter fetal insulin secretion or fetal insulin resistance strongly support the fetal insulin hypothesis (Table 1). These examples show how genetically determined alterations in pancreatic glucose sensing, insulin secretion or insulin resistance all have considerable effects on fetal growth. Insights have come from our new studies of mothers and neonates with mutations in the gene that codes for the glycolytic enzyme glucokinase, that acts as the 'pancreatic glucose sensor'[27]. Glucokinase gene mutation results in mild β-cell dysfunction with fasting blood glucose levels typically between 5.5–8 mmol/l; this hyperglycaemia is present in early childhood and shows little deterioration with age[28]. Figure 3 shows the effects of fetal and maternal mutations on mean birth weight centiles[29]. A mutation in the glucokinase gene in the mother resulted in a 601 g **increase** in fetal size mediated through increased fetal insulin secretion in response to maternal hyperglycaemia, but the same mutation in the fetus

Table 1 Single gene disorders that alter fetal insulin secretion or fetal insulin resistance

Condition	Genetic defect	Altered physiology	Birth weight
ALTERED INSULIN SECRETION			
Glucokinase deficiency	Heterozygous mutations in the glucokinase gene[52]	Reduced insulin secretion (to 30% of normal) resulting from reduced glucose sensing by the pancreas[53]	Reduced by 521 g compared to unaffected siblings[29]
Pancreatic agenesis	Homozygous mutation in IPF1 gene[32]	No fetal insulin secretion as a result of pancreatic agenesis	Markedly reduced below first centile[54]
Transient neonatal diabetes	Paternal disomy or duplication of 6q22-q23[34,55]	Markedly reduced insulin secretion Mechanism uncertain	Markedly reduced most <1st centile[35]
Nesideoblastosis	Homozygous mutation in the SUR or Kir6 genes[36,37]	Increased insulin secretion as a result of activation of the SUR receptor	Increased most >90th centile[38]
ALTERED INSULIN RESISTANCE			
Leprechaun syndrome	Homozygous mutation in the insulin receptor[56]	Marked insulin resistance	Markedly reduced most <1st centile[33]

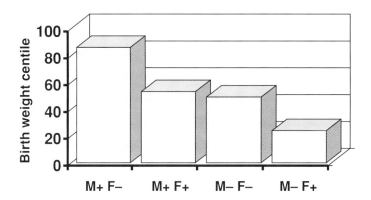

Fig. 3 The effect of mutations in the glucokinase gene on centile birth weight. Data from 58 offspring of parents with glucokinase mutations[29].

resulted in a 533 g **decrease** in its weight by reducing fetal insulin secretion. When both mother and fetus had the glucokinase mutation, the two opposing effects cancelled out and the baby was of normal weight[29].

Further examples of genes affecting fetal growth include the insulin promoter factor-1 (IPF-1) gene. This gene is crucial for normal pancreatic development and β-cell specific expression of the insulin gene[30,31]. Homozygous mutations result in pancreatic agenesis and greatly reduced fetal growth (<1st centile)[32]. Mutations in the insulin receptor result in marked insulin resistance and also greatly reduce fetal growth (<1st centile)[33]. Transient neonatal diabetes mellitus (TNDM) results from alterations to the imprinted pattern of a gene on chromosome 6[34]. Paternal disomy (the inheritance of two paternal chromosomes and none from the mother) or paternal duplication of this region results in two copies of this gene being expressed instead of one and, in addition to the diabetic phenotype, infants show reduced birth weight (most <1st centile)[35].

Homozygous mutations of the β-cell potassium channel sulphonylurea or Kir6 genes result in marked over-secretion of insulin for given glucose levels and cause persistent hypoglycaemia and hyperinsulinaemia in infants[36,37]. In keeping with the key role of insulin in fetal growth, these individuals are born at greatly increased birth size (>90th centile)[38].

X-chromosome abnormalities also result in low birth weight – a study of 14 females with either partial X chromosome deletions or X/autosome translocations demonstrated that those with a chromosome breakpoint proximal of Xq22 had low birth weight (<3 kg) and adult height (<155 cm)[39]. Interestingly, this region of the X-chromosome harbours the insulin receptor substrate-4 (IRS-4) gene (http://www.ncbi.nlm.nih.gov/genemap99/) an important component of the insulin-signalling pathway. IRS genes are crucial for normal growth and glucose homeostasis in mice[40]. Whether the reduced birth weight in X-chromosome deleted females is due to the loss of IRS-4 is not yet known.

Imprinted genes and growth

Genes that are imprinted play a critical role in growth. For the vast majority of human genes, two copies are required – one from the maternal and one from the paternal chromosome. The exceptions are imprinted genes in which either the maternal or paternal copy is

Table 2 Defects in imprinted genes resulting in alterations in growth

Condition	Genetic defect(s)	Effect on growth
Prader-Willi syndrome	Paternal deletion of 15q11-q13, maternal uniparental disomy of 15q11-q13	Mild prenatal growth retardation with a mean birth weight of 2.8-kg at term. Diminished growth in the majority of infants. Relatively increased body fat even in underweight children. (OMIM#176270)
Beckwith-Weidemann	Paternal duplication or paternal uniparental disomy of chromosome 11p15.5 resulting in biallelic expression of IGF-II	Generalised overgrowth – increased birth weight, exophalos, macroglossia, predisposition to embryonal tumours, in particular Wilms tumour (OMIM#130650)
Transient neonatal diabetes	Paternal uniparental disomy or duplication of 6q22-q23[34,55]	Reduced birth weight (most < 1st centile)[35] due to reduced insulin secretion. Gene unknown
Russell-Silver syndrome	Maternal duplication or maternal uniparental disomy of 7p11-p13 resulting in bi-allelic expression of GRB10 (growth factor receptor-bound protein)[57]	Prenatal and postnatal growth retardation including low birth weight possibly due to binding of GRB10 to the insulin receptor and the insulin-like growth factor I receptor and inhibition of the associated tyrosine kinase activity that is involved in the growth-promoting activities of insulin, IGF1 and IGFII (OMIM#180860)

inactivated in the parental gametes. Over 40 imprinted genes have been localised[41], and often this discovery has been facilitated by defects in imprinted genes resulting in a clinical syndrome. Notably, many of these syndromes result in abnormal patterns of growth, including alterations to birth size. Table 2 shows some of the defects involving imprinted genes and their effects on growth. The best characterised of these is Beckwith-Weidemann syndrome. This disorder is the result of paternal duplication or paternal uniparental disomy of a region of chromosome 11. The disease is thought to arise as a result of the expression of two rather than one paternal copy of IGF-II. IGF-II is imprinted with only the paternal copy being expressed in most tissues and has growth and metabolic effects mediated by the IGF-I receptor and insulin receptor[42,43].

Paternal diabetes reduces birth weight and predisposes to type 2 diabetes

Genetic defects in the glucokinase and Beckwith-Weidemann genes resulting in the syndromes described are very rare and cannot explain the association between birth weight and type 2 diabetes seen in the normal population. However, recent elegant studies in the Pima Indians strongly support the hypothesis that more common gene variants can explain the association between type 2 diabetes and reduced birth weight.

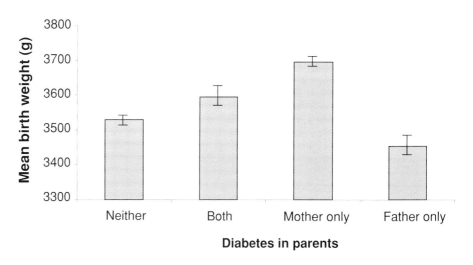

Fig. 4 Birth weight and parental diabetes in Arizona Pima-Indians. Values are expressed as means ± SE. General effect of parental diagnosis of diabetes on birth weight (P <0.001). Independent effect of maternal diabetes (P <0.001) and independent effect of paternal diabetes (P <0.001)[44]. [Reproduced with permission of *Diabetes*.]

Lindsay *et al* hypothesised that if genes were important in the link between birth size and type 2 diabetes, then low birth weight would be associated with paternal diabetes. If, however, intra-uterine environmental factors predominated, birth weight should be independent of paternal diabetes[44]. This study was possible because the Pima Indians of Arizona have one of the highest prevalences of type 2 diabetes in the world[45]; of 1608 subjects with birth weight data available 41% of fathers and 50% of mothers were diabetic[44]. The results strongly supported a role for genes; infants born to couples in which the father alone had diabetes were significantly lighter at birth than if mother, both, or neither of the parents had diabetes (Fig. 4). The most obvious explanation for this is that diabetes susceptibility genes inherited from the father are also affecting insulin-mediated growth. In support of this, the children with a diabetic father who were in the lowest tertile of birth weight were significantly more likely to be diabetic than those in the middle and highest tertiles[44].

This study also confirmed a key role for the intra-uterine environment. The offspring of mothers who were diagnosed as having diabetes, were heavier and had an increased risk of diabetes in latter life[44]. This is in keeping with previous studies in this population suggesting that exposure to hyperglycaemia *in utero* predisposes to diabetes. The 'U'-shaped curve seen with risk of diabetes in the Pima Indians[45] can now be explained by the increased risk of developing diabetes of small babies who have diabetic fathers and large babies who have diabetic mothers.

Genes influencing normal variation in birth weight

The recent data from the Pima Indian study strongly indicate that paternal, and therefore genetic, effects are important in normal variation in birth weight and that at least some of these genes may predispose to diabetes. But which genes are important? Several gene variants have recently been associated with alterations in birth size. Dunger *et al* demonstrated that the insulin VNTR is associated with altered birth weight, but only in infants that remained on the same post-natal growth rank from 0–2 years old[46]. Conversely, Casteels *et al* demonstrated an associated between birth size and a mitochondrial DNA variant, but only in infants that changed post-natal growth rank[47]. In addition, two recent studies have demonstrated associations between features of fetal and maternal metabolism, including birth size, and a DNA variant in the gene encoding a member of the important G-protein family of signal-transducing proteins[48,49]. Of these gene associations, the insulin VNTR is perhaps the most convincing. The insulin VNTR is also linked with type 2 diabetes but in a paternally specific manner[14]. This suggests the imprinted IGF-II gene, expression of which is partly controlled by the insulin VNTR[50],

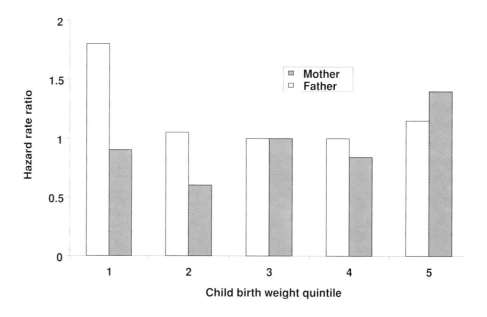

Fig. 5 Hazard rate ratio (mean and 95% CI) for later diabetes in parents who did not have diabetes at the time of birth of their children. Rates are compared to middle quintile of child birth weight which is set to 1. Birth weight quintile acted as a significant predictor of later paternal diabetes ($P < 0.005$)[44]. [Reproduced with permission of *Diabetes.*]

may influence both type 2 diabetes and birth weight, most obviously through its effects on growth and metabolism mediated by IGF-1 and insulin receptors. Further studies are required to investigate this.

Dissecting the genetics of birth weight and type 2 diabetes

If a common gene variant was found to influence both susceptibility to type 2 diabetes and birth weight, it would lend substantial weight to the argument that genes may explain the association between birth weight and adult disorders of metabolism. However, a number of hurdles lie in the way of this seemingly straightforward experiment. The first is that finding type 2 diabetes gene variants is very difficult due to the highly heterogeneous nature of the disease and poor understanding of the primary physiological defects. There are likely to be many genes all having subtle effects on diabetes risk and, therefore, very large and well characterised patient cohorts are needed. When we have a diabetes gene variant, how will it influence fetal growth? We know that maternal glucose levels influence fetal size as increased levels are correlated with increased fetal growth. However, a mother's blood glucose level is likely to be influenced by a number of factors including a conglomerate of genes that affect insulin secretion and action. Half of these genes she will pass to her fetus. As previously pointed out, therefore, a baby with a high future genetic risk of diabetes may be born large if inheriting most diabetes-risk genes from the mother or small if inheriting most diabetes-risk genes from the father[51]. This point is illustrated by the findings in Pima Indians that low birth weight is associated with an increased risk of paternal diabetes and high birth weight is associated with an increased risk of maternal diabetes (Fig. 5)[44].

Studies of putative diabetes genes on the effects of birth weight will, therefore, require careful characterisation of maternal glucose levels in addition to controlling for well known influences on birth weight such as gestational age, sex and maternal smoking. Only then are the effects of any single genetic factor likely to be detected.

Acknowledgements

We thank all our colleagues in Exeter and Professor Mark McCarthy for helpful discussion. Dr Tim Frayling is supported by the NHS South and West Research and Development Directorate. Figures 4 and 5 were reproduced with kind permission from *Diabetes*.

References

1   Barker DJP, Bull AR, Osmond C, Simmonds SJ. Fetal and placental size and risk of hypertension in adult life. *BMJ* 1990; **301**: 259–62
2   Barker DJP, Godfrey KM, Osmond C, Bull A. The relation of fetal length, ponderal index and head circumference to blood pressure and the risk of hypertension in adult life. *Paediatr Perinat Epidemiol* 1992; **6**: 35–44
3   Hales CN, Barker DJP, Clark PMS *et al.* Fetal and infant growth and impaired glucose tolerance at age 64. *BMJ* 1991; **303**: 1019–22
4   Hattersley AT, Tooke JE. The fetal insulin hypothesis: an alternative explanation of the association of low birth weight with diabetes and vascular disease. *Lancet* 1999; **353**: 1789–92
5   Vogler GP, McClearn GE, Snieder H *et al.* Genetics and behavioral medicine: risk factors for cardiovascular disease. *Behav Med* 1997; **22**: 141–9
6   Kobberling J, Tillil H. Empirical risk figures for first degree relatives of non-insulin-dependent diabetics. In: Kobberling J, Tattersall R. (eds) *The Genetics of Diabetes Mellitus*. London: Academic Press, 1982; 201–10
7   Risch N. Linkage strategies for genetically complex traits. I. Multilocus models. *Am J Hum Genet* 1990; **46**: 222–8
8   Rich SS. Mapping genes in diabetes: genetic epidemiological perspective. *Diabetes* 1990; **39**: 1315–9
9   Newman B, Selby JV, King MC, Slemenda C, Fabsitz R, Friedman GD. Concordance for type 2 (non-insulin-dependent) diabetes mellitus in male twins. *Diabetologia* 1987; **30**: 763–8
10 Serjeantson SW, Zimmet P. Genetics of NIDDM: pilgrim's progress. In: Alberti KGMM, Mazze RS. (eds) *Frontiers of Diabetes Research: Non-Insulin-Dependent Diabetes Mellitus*. Amsterdam: Elsevier, 1989; 21–36

11   Serjeantson SW, Owerbach D, Zimmet P, Nerup J, Thoma K. The genetics of diabetes in Nauru: effects of foreign admixture, HLA antigens and the insulin-gene-linked polymorphism. *Diabetologia* 1983; **25**: 13–7

12   Williams RC, Long JC, Hanson RL, Sievers ML, Knowler WC. Individual estimates of European genetic admixture associated with lower body-mass index, plasma glucose, and prevalence of type 2 diabetes in Pima Indians. *Am J Hum Genet* 2000; **66**: 527–38

13   Horikawa Y, Oda N, Cux NJ *et al*. Genetic variation in the calpain 10 gene (CAPN10) is associated with type 2 diabetes mellitus. *Nat Genet* 2000; 26(2): 163–75

14   Huxtable S, Saker P, Walker M *et al*. INS-VNTR dependent susceptibility to type 2 diabetes is mediated exclusively through paternally-transmitted class III alleles. *Diabetes* 2000; **49**: 126–30

15   Poulsen P, Vaag AA, Kyvik KO, Jensen MD, Beck-Nielsen H. Low birth weight is associated with NIDDM in discordant monozygotic and dizygotic twin pairs. *Diabetologia* 1997; **40**: 439–46

16   Godfrey KM, Barker DJ. Maternal birthweight and diet in pregnancy in relation to the infant's thinness at birth. *Br J Obstet Gynaecol* 1997; **104**: 663–7

17   Barkhouse KL, van Vleck LD, Cundiff LV, Buchanan DS, Marshall DM. Comparison of sire breed solutions for growth traits adjusted by mean expected progeny differences to a 1993 base. *J Anim Sci* 1998; **76**: 2287–93

18   Cundiff LV, MacNeil MD, Gregory KE, Koch RM. Between- and within-breed genetic analysis of calving traits and survival to weaning in beef cattle. *J Anim Sci* 1986; **63**: 27–33

19   Walton A, Hammond J. The maternal effects on growth and conformation in Shire horse–Shetland pony crosses. *Proc R Soc Lond B Biol Sci* 1938; 311–35

20   De Fronzo RA, Bonadonna RC, Ferrannini E. Pathogenesis of NIDDM: a balanced overview. *Diabetes Care* 1992; **15**: 318–68

21   Pederson J. Problems and Management. *The Pregnant Diabetic and Her New Born*. Baltimore, ND: Williams & Wilkins, 1977; 211–20

22   Naylor CD, Sermer M, Chen E, Sykora K. Cesarean delivery in relation to birth weight and gestational glucose tolerance: pathophysiology or practice style? Toronto Trihospital Gestational Diabetes Investigators. *JAMA* 1996; **275**: 1165–70

23   Tallarigo L, Giampietro O, Penno G, Miccoli R, Gregori G, Navalesi R. Relation of glucose tolerance to complications of pregnancy in non-diabetic women. *N Engl J Med* 1986; **315**: 989–92

24   Farmer G, Russell G, Hamilton-Nicol DR *et al*. The influence of maternal glucose metabolism on fetal growth, development and morbidity in 917 singleton pregnancies in non-diabetic women. *Diabetologia* 1988; **31**: 134–41

25   Breschi MC, Seghieri G, Bartolomei G, Gironi A, Baldi S, Ferrannini E. Relation of birthweight to maternal plasma glucose and insulin concentrations during normal pregnancy. *Diabetologia* 1993; **36**: 1315–21

26   Sermer M, Naylor CD, Gare DJ *et al*. Impact of increasing carbohydrate intolerance on maternal-fetal outcomes in 3637 women without gestational diabetes. The Toronto Tri-Hospital Gestational Diabetes Project. *Am J Obstet Gynecol* 1995; **173**: 146–56

27   Matschinsky F, Liang Y, Kesavan P *et al*. Glucokinase as pancreatic beta cell glucose sensor and diabetes gene. *J Clin Invest* 1993; **92**: 2092–8

28   Hattersley AT. Maturity-onset diabetes of the young: clinical heterogeneity explained by genetic heterogeneity. *Diabet Med* 1998; **15**: 15–24

29   Hattersley AT, Beards F, Ballantyne E, Appleton M, Harvey R, Ellard S. Mutations in the glucokinase gene of the fetus result in reduced birth weight. *Nat Genet* 1998; **19**: 268–70

30   Johnsson JL, Carlsson T, Edlund T, Edlund H. Insulin promoter factor 1 is required for pancreas development in mice. *Nature* 1994; **371**: 606–9

31   Ahlgren U, Jonsson J, Jonsson L, Simu K, Edlund H. Beta-cell-specific inactivation of the mouse Ipf1/Pdx1 gene results in loss of the beta-cell phenotype and maturity onset diabetes. *Genes Dev* 1998; **12**: 1763–8

32   Stoffers DA, Zinkin NT, Stanojevic V, Clarke WL, Habener JF. Pancreatic agenesis attributable to a single nucleotide deletion in the human IPF1 gene coding sequence. *Nat Genet* 1997; **15**: 106–10

33   Donohue WL, Uchida IA. Leprechaunism: a euphenism for a rare familial disorder. *J Pediatr* 1954; **45**: 505–19

34   Temple IK, Gardner RJ, Robinson DO *et al.* Further evidence for an imprinted gene for neonatal diabetes localised to chromosome 6q22-q23. *Hum Mol Genet* 1996; **5**: 1117–24

35   Shield JPH. Neonatal diabetes. In: Shield JPH, Baum JD. (eds) *Childhood Diabetes*, vol 4. London: Baillière Tindall, 1996; 681–740

36   Thomas PM, Cote GJ, Wohllk K *et al.* Mutations in the sulfonylurea receptor gene in familial persistent hyperinsulinemic hypoglycemia of infancy. *Science* 1995; **268**: 426–9

37   Thomas P, Ye Y, Lightner E. Mutation of the pancreatic islet inward rectifier Kir6.2 also leads to familial persistent hyperinsulinemic hypoglycemia of infancy. *Hum Mol Genet* 1996; **5**: 1809–12

38   Aparicio L, Carpenter MW, Schwartz R, Gruppuso PA. Prenatal diagnosis of familial neonatal hyperinsulinemia. *Acta Paediatr* 1993; **82**: 683–6

39   Maraschio P, Tupler R, Barbierato L *et al.* An analysis of Xq deletions. *Hum Genet* 1996; **97**: 375–81

40   Withers DJ, Gutierrez JS, Towery H *et al.* Disruption of IRS-2 causes type 2 diabetes in mice. *Nature* 1998; **391**: 900–3

41   Morison IM, Reeve AE. A catalogue of imprinted genes and parent-of-origin effects in humans and animals. *Hum Mol Genet* 1998; 7: 1599–609

42   Baker J, Liu J, Robertson E, Efstratiadis A. Role of insulin-like growth factors in embryonic and postnatal growth. *Cell* 1993; **75**: 73–82

43   Louvi A, Accili D, Efstratiadis A. Growth-promoting interaction of IGF-II with the insulin receptor during mouse embryonic development. *Dev Biol* 1997; **189**: 33–48

44   Lindsay RS, Dabelea D, Roumain J, Hanson RL, Bennett PH, Knowler WC. Type 2 diabetes and low birth weight. *Diabetes* 2000; **49**: 445–9

45   McCance DR, Pettitt DJ, Hanson RL, Jacobsson LT, Knowler WC, Bennett PH. Birth weight and non-insulin dependent diabetes: thrifty genotype, thrifty phenotype, or surviving small baby genotype? *BMJ* 1994; **308**: 942–5

46   Dunger DB, Ong KK, Huxtable SJ *et al.* Association of the INS VNTR with size at birth. ALSPAC Study Team. Avon Longitudinal Study of Pregnancy and Childhood. *Nat Genet* 1988; **19**: 98–100

47   Casteels K, Ong K, Phillips D *et al.* Mitochondrial 16189 variant, thinness at birth and type 2 diabetes. *Lancet* 1999; **353**: 1499–500

48   Gutersohn A, Naber C, Muller N, Erbel R, Siffert W. G protein b3 subunit 825TT genotype and post-pregnancy weight retention. *Lancet* 2000; **355**: 1240–1

49   Hocher B, Slowinski T, Stolze T, Pleschka A, Neumayer H-H, Halle H. Association of maternal G-protein subunit 825T allele with low birthweight. *Lancet* 2000; **355**: 1241–2

50   Paquette J, Giannoukakis N, Polychronakos C, Vafiadis P, Deal C. The INS 5' variable number of tandem repeats is associated with IGF2 expression in humans. *J Biol Chem* 1998; **273**: 14158–64

51   McCarthy M. Weighing in on diabetes risk. *Nat Genet* 1998; **19**: 209–10

52   Froguel P, Zouali H, Vionnet N *et al.* Familial hyperglycemia due to mutations in glucokinase. Definition of a subtype of diabetes mellitus. *N Engl J Med* 1993; **328**: 697–702

53   Byrne MM, Sturis J, Clement K *et al.* Insulin secretory abnormalities in subjects with hyperglycemia due to glucokinase mutations. *J Clin Invest* 1994; **93**: 1120–30

54   Wright NM, Metzger DL, Borowitz SM, Clarke WL. Permanent neonatal diabetes mellitus and pancreatic exocrine insufficiency resulting from congenital pancreatic agenesis. *Am J Dis Child* 1993; **147**: 607–9

55   Temple IK, James RS, Crolla JA *et al.* An imprinted gene(s) for diabetes? *Nat Genet* 1995; **9**: 110–2

56   Elsas LJ, Endo F, Strumlauf E, Elders J, Priest JH. Leprechaunism: an inherited defect in a high-affinity insulin receptor. *Am J Hum Genet* 1985; **37**: 73–88

57   Yoshihashi H, Maeyama K, Kosaki R *et al.* Imprinting of human GRB10 and its mutations in two patients with Russell-Silver syndrome. *Am J Hum Genet* 2000; **67**: 476–82

Animal models and programming of the metabolic syndrome

Caroline E Bertram and **Mark A Hanson**

Centre for Fetal Origins of Adult Disease, Princess Anne Hospital, Southampton, UK

The purpose of this review is to consider how current animal models of fetal programming contribute to knowledge of the metabolic syndrome in adult humans. Low birth weight infants have an increased risk of developing cardiovascular and coronary heart disease, hypertension, diabetes and stroke in adulthood. A number of animal studies confirm the association between events during fetal life and subsequent adult disease. This review considers how these have contributed to our understanding of this relationship, and how they may help to uncover the underlying mechanisms. The importance of dietary, pharmacological, genetic and surgical models is assessed, and their usefulness in the prevention of human disease evaluated. Although progress has been made, further investigations using animals are needed to clarify the mechanisms involved in the programming of adult disease. Once these processes are understood, it may be possible to identify and protect at-risk individuals.

Human epidemiological studies link the incidence of a number of adult diseases, such as type 2 diabetes, cardiovascular disease (CVD) and hypertension with poor prenatal nutrition and low birth weight. This group of diseases is often referred to under the term metabolic syndrome (syndrome X). The data relate low ponderal index or short body length to these diseases, suggesting that a compromised maternal–fetal nutrient supply results in fetal growth retardation. This in turn is linked to altered 'programming' of development of fetal organs and of physiological homeostatic control processes. As such, programming occurs during critical periods of development, changes become permanent and lead to later pathophysiological events. The mechanisms underlying the pathophysiology of these associations, however, have yet to be elucidated[1].

Despite the substantial epidemiological evidence for fetal origins of adult disease, there are intrinsic limitations in long-term retrospective studies. Some aspects can, however, be focused on by using the controlled conditions afforded by animal models, a number of which have been developed to study this *in utero* programming phenomenon. The purpose of this review is to compare current models, not only to summarise the

Correspondence to:
Prof. M Hanson, Centre
for Fetal Origins of Adult
Disease, Princess Anne
Hospital, Coxford Road,
Southampton
SO16 5AY, UK

data thus far accumulated, but also to consider future options for this area of research. At present, species studied include the rat, mouse, guinea pig, sheep and non-human primate, and treatments used include dietary, pharmacological, genetic and surgical manipulation.

A key determinant of fetal growth is the availability of protein. Through most of fetal life, amino acids, rather than glucose, determine insulin secretion by β-pancreatic cells[2], and this control of fetal insulin secretion links the availability of amino acids to support fetal growth with the rate of fetal growth since insulin is an important fetal growth hormone. Other nutrients, including oxygen, are critical for optimum fetal growth, and it is possible that a combination of deficiencies are involved in human fetal growth retardation. Research in many laboratories is directed towards disentangling the many threads in this complicated story. In some, an isocaloric maternal low protein (MLP) diet has been used to explore the mechanisms by which protein metabolism affects developing organs. Other studies have used varying degrees of global reduction in nutrition. Many studies have employed pharmacological methods, genetic manipulation or surgical techniques to produce useful animal models. These will be discussed briefly below. It is noteworthy that, in some of these studies, effects on the development of homeostatic mechanisms were produced even in the absence of body growth restriction – findings analogous to those in humans who were exposed to the Dutch famine (*see* Hales & Barker, this issue). It is, therefore, possible to envisage a spectrum of health problems in adult life deriving from the influence of the intra-uterine environment and maternal/placental/fetal compensatory responses to a diet mildly to severely altered in its composition or its volume. It is also important to note that even if an isocaloric low protein diet does not affect birth weight significantly in the first generation, it may reduce it in subsequent generations[3].

Dietary manipulation

The concept that maternal nutrition can programme adult disease was established in animal experiments. Over 30 years ago, Winick and Noble showed that poor nutrition during gestation led irreversibly to reduced cell number in tissues such as the pancreas[4]. In 1974, Weinkove *et al* established that permanent impairment of insulin secretion resulted from perinatal protein restriction[5], and subsequently post-weaning protein depletion was shown to produced the same result[6]. More recently, Snoeck and co-workers demonstrated that maternal protein deprivation caused reduced β-cell proliferation and islet size in the offspring[7].

Two different dietary strategies are used at present – global nutritional restriction, and isocaloric low protein manipulation – and these are discussed below.

Global undernutrition

A number of studies using different levels of global dietary restriction have been reported. In New Zealand, Gluckman's laboratory developed a rat model of IUGR using severe maternal dietary restriction (30% of *ad libitum*) throughout gestation and examined the effects of fetal growth retardation on the endocrine and metabolic status during the perinatal period[8]. Previous work had supplied evidence that there is a central role for fetal IGF-1 in the regulation of fetal growth, and that both maternal and fetal IGF-I are regulated by nutrient availability[9]. In the sheep, maternal administration of IGF-I has been shown to enhance amino acid and glucose uptake by the placenta and to promote glucose delivery to the fetus. In rat studies, maternal plasma IGF-I levels were significantly reduced throughout gestation, but not postnatally, and both the mean body weights of late gestation fetuses and the placental weights were significantly lower than controls. Taken together, these studies in the sheep and rat establish a link between IGF-1 and fetal growth. Interestingly, while plasma IGF-1 and plasma insulin levels in the pups were significantly reduced from birth to postnatal day 9, this did not persist into adulthood.

A less severe global restriction model was used by Holemans and co-workers who studied blood pressure (using an implanted femoral artery catheter) in female rats whose dams had received a 50% reduction in food intake in the second half of pregnancy. No significant difference in blood pressure was found, though small mesenteric arteries had reduced endothelium-dependent relaxation (to acetylcholine and bradykinin) but enhanced sensitivity to exogenous nitric oxide (sodium nitroprusside)[10]. This indicated that while reduced synthesis of nitric oxide and prostacyclin altered vascular function, it was insufficient to result in a change in blood pressure.

Even mild global restriction has been shown to produce alterations in both metabolism and the HPA axis. Studies in guinea pigs fed an 85% of *ad libitum* diet throughout pregnancy showed that maternal undernutrition and small size at birth permanently alter postnatal cholesterol homeostasis in the male offspring[11]. This is interesting because a number of investigations into CVD susceptibility indicate that prenatal and early postnatal manipulation of cholesterol affect adult cholesterol metabolism in rodents and baboons[12]. In the sheep, a 15% global reduction of total diet during the first half of pregnancy resulted in blunted ACTH and cortisol responses to exogenous CRH and AVP administration (d113–116 and 125–127), and also a reduced cortisol response to ACTH[13]. When maternal food reduction was followed by acute hypoxemic challenges between days 114–129, plasma ACTH and cortisol responses were also reduced relative to controls. In both studies, basal plasma and cortisol responses were unaltered[14], suggesting that the effects are predominantly manifest on the response of the HPA axis to endogenous and exogenous stimuli. It is interesting to note that even the mildest maternal global undernutrition has significant effects at two or more levels of the axis.

Maternal low protein (MLP)

Maternal low protein models of fetal programming have been extensively used to study the mechanisms that link maternal nutrition with impaired fetal growth and later cardiovascular disease and diabetes. Interestingly, the differing composition of the low protein diets used in individual laboratories, while generally causing low birth weight, appear to predispose the offspring to different pathophysiological effects in adulthood. A direct comparison of two of these diets in relation to their ability to cause hypertension in adults was recently undertaken by Langley-Evans[15], *viz* the diet used at Southampton and the Hope Farm diet used by Hales and colleagues in Cambridge and by others[16]. While the diets differed in their overall fat content, fatty acid composition, methionine content and the source of carbohydrate, the protocols used were identical. It was found that offspring of rats fed the Southampton diet, but not those on the Hope Farm diet, became hypertensive. Langley-Evans concluded that different low protein diet manipulations (at 8–9%) in rat pregnancy elicit different programming effects, and that the balance of protein with other nutrients may be a critical determinant of the long-term health effects of maternal undernutrition in pregnancy.

It is not clear how restricted maternal protein supply perturbs fetal growth. In the rat there are two phases of protein metabolism during pregnancy. During the anabolic phase, maternal body protein is accumulated which can then be used to support fetal growth during the catabolic phase. However, it is not yet known whether this mechanism can compensate for reduced dietary protein intake and thus maintain the supply of free amino acids to the fetus. Analysis of free amino acids in fetuses and mothers fed 9% casein diets showed a reduction in maternal threonine which was not evident either in control rats or in non-pregnant rats fed the low protein diet[17]. Rees *et al* suggest that the threonine-methionine-homocysteine group of amino acids may lead to adverse effects in the protein-deficient mother and her offspring. However, although the 9% casein diet supplies insufficient protein for a pregnant rat, this percentage lies within normal nutritional parameters for a non-pregnant rat. While Rees's conclusions may be valid, the results should be tested against a nutritionally challenged non-pregnant control.

Maternal protein restriction affects islet cells, as well as insulin-sensitive tissues such as liver, muscle, adipocytes, kidney and brain in the offspring[15]. Protein availability appears to have a specific role in the development of fetal β-cells. *In vitro*, increased essential amino acid concentrations amplify fetal β-cell differentiation, multiplication and insulin secretion more efficiently than increased glucose concentration. Abnormal features thus acquired by the developing β-cell may then lead to postnatal pathological events[18]. Feeding an isocaloric low protein diet during gestation alters the profile of amino acids in maternal and fetal plasma as well as in amniotic fluid, though neither the total essential and non-essential amino acid concentrations nor the glucose and insulin levels are modified. α-Amino-butyric acid, phosphoserine, taurine and valine are reduced in maternal as well as in fetal plasma[19]. Kwong *et al* investigated the effect of mild protein malnourishment on pre-implantation embryos, and found that feeding 9% protein to mothers from conception to implantation only, followed by standard chow, resulted in offspring which developed hypertension as adults. These embryos displayed significantly reduced cell numbers, induced by a slower rate of cellular proliferation rather than by increased apoptosis. At day 4, insulin and essential amino acids in maternal serum were reduced, compared to controls, whilst glucose levels were increased[20]. These changes in maternal values may provide one or more of the mechanisms by which altered maternal diet produces signals for the early embryo.

Maternal protein deprivation studies have also shown uneven distribution of islet cell proliferation in the endocrine pancreas, and islet cell size, pancreatic insulin content and islet vascular density were all reduced at birth. Additionally, when the low protein diet was maintained during weaning, the ontogeny of the endocrine pancreas of offspring was disturbed in that there were more apoptotic cells in islets while the number of cells positive for IGF-II, a survival factor preventing apoptosis, was decreased[21]. In fetal β-cells, insulin secretion was halved *in vitro*, while *in vivo* offspring with normal glucose, insulin and amino acid profiles reacted abnormally to a glucose challenge[22]. Insulin levels were low before and during pregnancy, but plasma glucose levels were higher than normal.

When the adult offspring were maintained on a low protein diet postnatally, they had an abnormal amino acid profile, a smaller endocrine pancreas and reduced pancreatic insulin content. Additionally, there was a reduction in islet blood vessel density together with pancreatic and islet blood flow. Interestingly, the islet mitochondria had reduced glycero-phosphate dehydrogenase (mGPDH) activity[7]. This reduction is also observed in islet cells of human subjects with type 2 diabetes[23].

Intergenerational studies show that reduced birth weight continues through subsequent generations. After an oral glucose challenge, pregnant offspring had low plasma insulin and high plasma glucose levels and their pups had more marked differences in plasma insulin, insulin content and endocrine pancreas density than the previous generation[23]. A similar intergenerational effect of a protein restricted diet has already been observed on brain development and tryptophan metabolism[24].

In the liver, the MLP diet causes changes in zonation and enzyme activity, including a reduction in glucokinase and an increase in PEPCK activity, and altered regulation of hepatic glucose output[25], which are not restored at adulthood even when the animals are fed a normal diet[26]. Insulin receptor number was increased in the liver, skeletal muscle and white fat adipocytes[27]. Additionally, the adipocytes were smaller and did not show changes in GLUT4 expression, although this was increased in the plasma membrane of skeletal muscle[28]. The adipocytes of adults had a greater glucose uptake and a higher phosphatidylinositol 3-kinase activity[29]. Adipose tissue of offspring was also affected by global dietary restriction, which comprises low protein availability in the dams. In this instance, white adipose tissue increased and brown adipose tissue decreased in the adult, possibly indicating lower sympathetic activity. Rats whose mothers had restricted food during the first 2 weeks of pregnancy indeed became obese; but, depending on the strain and the diet used, it was either the males or the females which were affected[30,31]

Hoet and colleagues in Louvain demonstrated that protein plays a key role in development of the islets of Langerhans *in utero*. Offspring of rats fed a diet containing 50% less protein during pregnancy had poor β-cell proliferative capacity and islet size at birth, as well as reduced blood vessel density in the islets[32]. Rats which were weaned on a low protein diet for 3 weeks also had a permanently altered insulin response to glucose. MLP offspring fed a low protein diet into adulthood were subsequently shown to have reduced glucose tolerance associated with reduced insulin secretion. Interestingly, the MLP group fed normal chow after birth had an intermediate response[33]. This suggests that exposure to poor nutrition over brief periods during development, even when followed by normal food intake, can lead to irreversible changes. Thus, the developing pancreas appears to be sensitive to amino acid availability, and its endocrine function may also be regulated by nutritional elements. Consistent with the above findings are Hales' observations on pancreatic glucokinase, an enzyme which plays a central role in the regulation of glucose-stimulated insulin release from the β-cell (glucose enters β-cell via GLUT2 transporter protein and is then phosphorylated by glucokinase). Glucokinase activity was measured in whole pancreatic extracts, and compared to offspring of control and MLP dams which were cross-fostered. MLP offspring were found to have significantly lower pancreatic glucokinase activity compared with controls and crossover groups. Using the same model, Hales and colleagues looked at glucose tolerance. All rats became less glucose tolerant with age, but the worsening of glucose tolerance was more profound in the MLP group. Males tended to have higher plasma insulin concentrations, suggesting that, as in the human condition, the glucose intolerance was due mainly to insulin resistance. In females the situation appeared to be reversed, suggesting that their lower glucose tolerance was due mainly to insulin deficiency[15].

High fat diet in pregnancy

In addition to the phenomena obtained by undernutrition, studies of Pima Indians suggest that prenatal overnutrition can also programme later susceptibility to type 2 diabetes[34], and there is evidence that dietary fat intake during pregnancy increases the prevalence of cardiovascular risk factors in children[35]. Offspring of rats fed high saturated fats during pregnancy have fetal insulin resistance[36], abnormal cholesterol metabolism[37] and raised adult blood pressure[38]. These symptoms would certainly predispose offspring to obesity in adulthood, and it is possible that a high fat diet in childhood or adulthood would amplify their effects.

Eriksson and colleagues conducted a longitudinal study of catch-up growth and death from CVD in Helsinki, and found that the highest death rates occurred in men who were thin at birth, but whose weight caught up, so that they had an average or above average body mass from the age of 7 years. They concluded that death from CVD might be a consequence of poor prenatal nutrition followed by improved postnatal nutrition[39]. In consequence, a number of laboratories are now investigating the effect of cafeteria diets on offspring which were malnourished *in utero* and the results are awaited with interest.

Blood pressure measurement

There has been much debate recently regarding the measurement of blood pressure in the rat and this merits discussion here. Blood pressure can be measured using one of three methods:

1 Many studies, including those performed at Southampton and Cambridge use the indirect tail-cuff plethysmography method, which involves restraint and mild heat stress to vasodilate the tail bed. Only systolic pressure can be reliably measured and the method gives a single point measurement.

2 An in-dwelling carotid or iliac artery catheter allows continuous measurements of diastolic, systolic and pulse pressures to be taken with minimal disturbance, though the fact that the animal is continuously attached to a cable is inherently stressful. The catheter must be implanted under general anaesthesia, and the time taken to recover cannot be clearly established.

3 Most recently, it has been possible to use radiotelemetric methods which utilise an in-dwelling catheter in the descending aorta coupled to an intraperitoneal transmitter. This method has the benefit of a stress-free environment and the opportunity for 24 h monitoring of diastolic, systolic and pulse pressures.

The hypertensive model produced by mild protein malnutrition developed at Southampton has provided consistent data from a number of different laboratories, using tail cuff plethysmography. Experience has shown that providing the rat is trained with this equipment, stress can be kept to a minimum. These data have been reproduced when blood pressure was measured by cannulation in anaesthetized rats[40], but it is important now to validate these results using the latest telemetric methods, and this is presently being undertaken. Using telemetry, Tonkiss *et al* found only small baseline changes in diastolic pressure, with an augmented elevation of systolic and diastolic pressures when the animal was subjected to stress, and they questioned the validity of the larger elevations in blood pressure in MLP offspring observed using the tail-cuff procedure[41]. However, this study utilised a diet which differed not only in protein content (6%) but also in fat source, mineral balance and methionine levels. Since it has been demonstrated that different diets produce differing effects on blood pressure (see above)[15], a similar study using the Southampton diet is underway to clarify the situation. Additionally, the stress used by Tonkiss was olfactory (ammonia) and this may elicit a different response to that caused by restraint stress. The topic of the stress response is discussed later.

Pharmacological manipulation

Streptozotocin

The most common pharmacological model for diabetes in rodents and sheep is the administration of streptozotocin (STZ). It is mostly used as a tool for elucidating mechanisms which result from induction of the disease directly in the experimental animal. However, some studies have employed STZ to investigate programming of diabetes, and as such it has a place in this review (see also van Assche *et al*, this issue). Mild, maternal diabetes induced by STZ increased birth weight, produced β-cell hyperplasia in pancreatic endocrine tissue and an increase in the number of degranulated cells. However, when severe diabetes was induced, the fetal weight, islet size and β-cell mass were decreased. Additionally, in STZ-induced maternal diabetes, the pups of a second generation showed a reduction in birth weight together with permanent changes in endocrine pancreatic structure and function. Pups from both groups became diabetic at adulthood[42]. Pancreatic insulin depletion in pups from moderately diabetic dams and insulin resistance in pups from severely diabetic mothers were causal in initiating the diabetes in the offspring postnatally[43]. Additionally, maternal STZ-induced diabetes affected the responses of small resistance arteries in the pups[44].

Pharmacological disruption of the glucocorticoid pathway

A great deal of work has been targeted at glucocorticoid exposure in the fetus and at glucocorticoid receptor (GR) status both *in utero* and in adult life. Goland *et al* found 5-fold higher corticotrophin releasing hormone (CRH) concentrations in cord blood plasma of growth-retarded babies, suggesting an overactive fetal HPA axis in pregnancies associated with growth retardation. Furthermore, this increased activity appears to be permanent as adult hypertensive patients demonstrated increased sensitivity to cortisol in dermal vasoconstriction tests[45]. Many of the phenotypic features of the metabolic syndrome are also seen in Cushing's disease, suggesting that antagonism of the effects of insulin by increased glucocorticoid hormone action may occur in patients with the syndrome. However, increasing evidence suggests that the HPA axis is not grossly altered in these individuals. For example, cortisol concentrations are usually increased in patients with Cushing's disease but are decreased in patients with the metabolic syndrome[46,47]. Interestingly, Phillips *et al* found that plasma cortisol concentrations were increased (although still in the normal range) in men whose birth weights were low (<5.5 kg) compared with those who weighed >9.5 kg, a trend that was independent of age and body mass index. This suggests that plasma concentrations of cortisol within the normal range could have an important effect on blood pressure and glucose tolerance and provides evidence that intra-uterine programming of the HPA axis may be a mechanism underlying the association between low birth weight and the insulin resistance syndrome in adult life[48].

There is some evidence that HPA axis function in MLP offspring is modified resulting in hypersensitivity to glucocorticoid actions. While plasma corticosterone concentrations are similar at all points of the light cycle in rats exposed to control or MLP diets *in utero*, the normal diurnal variation in ACTH secretion was absent in the rats exposed to low protein, suggesting the adrenal response to ACTH is altered. The increased sensitivity to glucocorticoids (GC) action in the absence of elevated hormone concentrations may be mediated at the level of receptor binding. MLP rats have increased GR numbers in a variety of tissues[49,50], and the up-regulation of receptors in MLP animals may increase sensitivity and amplify the actions of circulating and tissue corticosterone.

Glucocorticoids induce the expression of numerous genes. During fetal life, the expression of many of these genes at the correct developmental stage is essential for optimal maturation of tissues. Normally, exposure to glucocorticoid does not occur until late gestation when cortisol (human, ovine) or corticosterone (rat) is produced by the fetal adrenal. It has been shown in the rat that if placental 11β-hydroxysteroid dehydrogenase 2 (11β-HSD2) activity is reduced, maternal glucocorticoid can cross the placenta inappropriately, and modify the HPA axis[56]. We have shown recently that the MLP rat offspring have higher levels of glucocorticoid receptor in adulthood and that this increase is tissue specific[52]. Langley-Evans showed that the MLP rat model has reduced placental 11β-HSD2, suggesting that excessive maternal glucocorticoids are transferred to the fetus, possibly permanently altering the set point of the HPA axis[56]. McMillen and co-workers found that while 11β-HSD2 was differentially regulated in the fetal adrenal and kidney in the sheep fetus during late gestation, expression was not affected by placental growth restriction. Expression of hepatic 11β-HSD1 mRNA, which is normally increased in the second half of pregnancy was enhanced (2-fold) by placental growth restriction[53], suggesting that there is increased hepatic exposure to cortisol in the growth-restricted fetus, which may be important in the reprogramming of hepatic physiology that occurs after growth restriction *in utero*. Strong evidence for this comes from pharmacological studies. Studies using the synthetic glucocorticoid dexamethasone (DEX), and the 11β-HSD inhibitor carbenoxolone (CBX) demonstrated that failure to inactivate maternal glucocorticoid by fetal and placental 11β-HSD2 gives rise to rats with features of the metabolic syndrome[54,55]. This effect could be prevented by administration of metyrapone (11β hydroxylase inhibitor) which blocked the synthesis of corticosteroids by both mother and fetus. Expression of glucocorticoid-sensitive genes, such as phosphoenolpyruvate carboxykinase (PEPCK) is also altered in the offspring, suggesting that the changes made to GC and GR *in utero* have effects on the metabolic efficiency of the offspring, leading to type 2 diabetes and other symptoms of the metabolic syndrome. Work undertaken in Jonathan Seckl's laboratory has focused on the HPA axis, using DEX or CBX. Administration of i.v. CBX during pregnancy led to hyperglycaemia in offspring, suggesting that inappropriate maternal glucocorticoid in the fetal circulation may be a factor in the programming of type 2 diabetes. 11β-HSD2 is normally co-located with the mineralocorticoid receptor (MR), and confers selectivity by inactivation of glucocorticoids which would otherwise bind to the MR. Interestingly, in sheep, CBX is a less potent inhibitor of 11β-HSD2 than in other species[58].

When rats were exposed to the DEX in late gestation, hepatic PEPCK and GR expression were permanently altered, causing glucose intolerance in adult offspring[55]. Unlike endogenous glucocorticoid, DEX is able to cross the placenta without being inactivated by placental 11β-HSD2[59]. When fetal sheep were exposed to DEX for 2 days at d27/150 they became hypertensive in adulthood, while those exposed at d64/150 did not. This programming was independent of insulin resistance or amino acid metabolism, but the DEX exposure did lead to increased insulin sensitivity of the inhibition of lipolysis, which may increase susceptibility to the development of obesity postnatally[60]. Clearly gluco-corticoids exert powerful effects on development at specific times, and these merit further investigation.

Genetic models

Recently, it has become apparent that the spontaneously hypertensive rat (SHR) strain is somewhat more than a purely genetic model of hyper-tension. Like the infants identified in a number of studies of human populations in the UK and world-wide[1], SHR pups are born small with a large associated placenta. A series of studies by McCarty and colleagues has demonstrated that cross-fostering of SHR offspring with normo-tensive dams prevents development of hypertension. This effect has a clear critical window in the early postnatal period and appears to involve a nutritional, rather than a behavioural stimulus, since SHR milk has an altered electrolyte balance, is low in protein and has a different fatty acid profile when compared to Wistar Kyoto rat milk[61].

The recent development of a maternal low protein mouse model (personal communication by CB Whorwood) will allow mice to be used in studies focusing on particular genes of interest. For example, IGF-I[63] knockout mice, IGF-II transgenic mice[64], IRS-1 disrupted mice[65], and tissue-specific insulin receptor knockout mice[66] could be used to pinpoint the mechanisms involved in programming of insulin resistance/glucose intolerance. Equally, mice with disruptions of the HPA axis such as CRH-deficiency[67] could be used to test the hypotheses implicating changes in the fetal HPA axis set-point.

Surgical models

Surgical interventions have been used primarily to provide further evidence of phenomena found in dietary or pharmacological models of programming. For example, adrenalectomy in the rat[40,54] was used in conjunction with synthetic glucocorticoid administration to confirm that maternal glucocorticoids are involved in the programming of hyper-tension in the offspring: adult female rats that had been adrenalectomized prior to mating and fed low protein diets during pregnancy gave birth to normotensive offspring, whilst administration of DEX to adrenalect-omized rats re-instated the hypertensive phenotype[40].

Disruption to fetal nutrition via the placenta can be achieved using a number of procedures, such as carunclectomy, placental embolisation and uterine artery ligation. Persson and Jansson ligated the arterial supply to one uterine horn in guinea pigs, which produced growth retardation of the pups in that horn whilst pups from the untreated horn were unaffected. The pups from the ligated horn had higher blood pressure than their litter-mates, although very severe reductions of birth weight (50–60%) were required to produce 10 mmHg increase in blood pressure. This work showed that nutritional deprivation during fetal life led to a reduction is tissue cell number which could not be reversed by adequate postnatal nutrition[68]. In a more recent study using telemetry, however, they found no correlation between blood pressure and birth weight[69]. In the sheep, it is relatively easy to undertake fetal as well as maternal manipulations. Removal of endometrial caruncles prior to conception (carunclectomy) has been used to manipulate fetal and placental growth rate. This procedure produces fetuses that are up to half normal size, albeit with a high incidence of mortality/fetal re-absorbtion, and the reduced placental size causes a fall in placental transport capacity which has significant consequences for the fetus. Decreased fetal growth velocity, soft tissue wasting and low birth weight are seen, with increased morbidity and mortality perinatally, and increased risk of pathophysiological effects on the cardiovascular system as well as type 2 diabetes in adulthood[70].

Murotsuki and colleagues embolised the fetal side of the placenta and measured cardiovascular and hormonal changes in fetal heart. They concluded that, as a result of fetal hypoxaemia and increased umbilical artery resistance caused by chronic placental damage, fetuses developed arterial hypertension and asymmetrical growth restriction, as well as myocardial hypertrophy due to increased afterload to the heart and raised plasma noradrenaline[71]. Using the same technique, this group also found that chronic hypoxaemia selectively inhibited renal 11β-HSD2 mRNA expression and enzyme activity in the ovine fetus, contributing, at least in part, to the mechanisms leading to fetal hypertension[72].

Which models relate to human disease?

Animal models allow study of the pathophysiology of disease, and afford a means to study the underlying biochemical and molecular biological mechanisms. Whilst they cannot be used entirely as a substitute for the study of human diabetes, they allow exploration of aspects which cannot ethically be considered in the patient. A drawback is that the dietary model does not cause frank diabetes in the rat, although it does cause symptoms which are consistent with future manifestation of the disease.

All the approaches discussed provide methods for the elucidation of aspects of the programming phenomenon. Possibly, however, pharmacological, genetic and surgical manipulations should be regarded as tools for further understanding of the metabolic syndrome in the nutritional model.

On the face of it, global dietary restriction appears to have more relevance to the human condition than isocaloric low protein diets. Although both regimens produce effects equivalent to symptoms of the metabolic syndrome, an isocaloric diet is easier to manipulate in order to tease out underlying mechanisms[15]. However, it will also be important to study a diet that more closely mimics sub-optimal human nutrition to identify possible interventions. Equally important is the study of postnatal diet on a system which is already compromised by intra-uterine nutritional restriction. If a balanced diet during pregnancy is not achieved, a central question to be answered is whether postnatal nutritional or pharmacological intervention can prevent the adult disease. As alterations to the HPA axis are one of the most important features in programming of adult disease, research using the protein restricted model backed up by pharmacological work, best serves the purpose. This would permit interference with the stress axis at a number of levels and thus enable isolation of the relevant nutritional deficit. Equally, surgical intervention which reduces fetal nutrition can be used in conjunction with, or instead of, dietary manipulation in order to replicate the metabolic syndrome in offspring. It is particularly useful in larger animals, such as the sheep, since the outcome of any manipulation can be directly monitored in a viable fetus.

Though animal models manifest most symptoms associated with the metabolic syndrome, frank disease is not easily reproducible, and this could be a criticism of this *in vivo* research. However, a combination of dietary, pharmacological, genetic and surgical manipulations provide indicators of the disorders involved and as such are valuable tools in the elucidation of the role of programming *in utero* as a cause of adult disease.

Do the various models give a clue to finding a common path?

In this review, we have shown that the effects of fetal undernutrition are manifest at various levels, as summarized in Figure 1.

Epigenetic

Recent studies on imprinting give new insights into how changes in gene expression can determine the trajectory of fetal growth[73] and environmental conditions can produce effects on the early embryo[20]. The effect of diet on expression of some GC-sensitive proteins has been

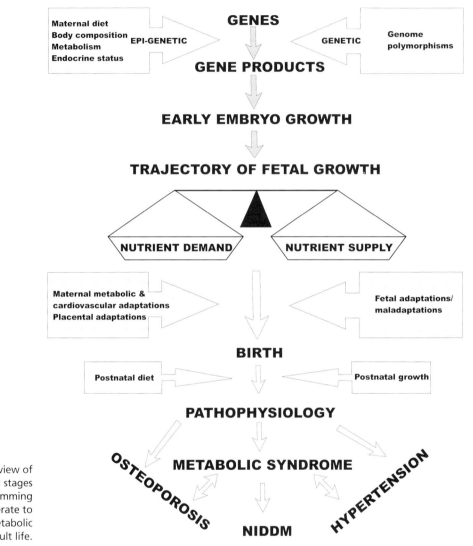

Fig. 1 Overview of developmental stages at which programming effects could operate to produce the metabolic syndrome in adult life.

established. For example, placental activity of 11β-HSD2 is reduced by maternal protein restriction. This enzyme plays a crucial role in the development of the fetal adrenal and hence may determine patterns of glucocorticoid secretion throughout life, and may alter fetal blood pressure through increased exposure to maternal glucocorticoids[48]. Hypertension induced by reduced maternal protein is abolished by inhibition of cortisol synthesis, leading to the hypothesis that maternal protein restriction programmes life-long changes in the fetal HPA axis and resets homeostatic mechanisms controlling blood pressure[23].

Limited protein intake during gestation leads to alterations in glucose output by the liver as well as in the sensitivity of tissues to insulin. Glucose transporters in muscles and the expression of key components of insulin signalling pathways in adipocytes are also altered. In addition, studies have suggested that maternal dietary restriction during gestation and lactation and transient dietary protein restriction after weaning may permanently alter growth hormone secretion in offspring[74]. In the sheep, the pituitary response to a CRH challenge and the adrenal cortical response to an ACTH challenge are reduced[75,76]. It is proposed that the suppression of the HPA axis function relates to prior exposure to elevated corticosteroids[38,77] and it is already known that DEX administration suppresses ovine HPA axis function[78].

Nutrient demand/nutrient supply

Both the experimental conditions of maternal protein restriction and diabetes stress the impact of maternal nutritional limitation or poor health in producing effects on the offspring. An isocaloric low protein diet during pregnancy reduces the fetal:placental weight ratio, produces elevated systolic blood pressure in the offspring and produces changes in glutathione metabolism and glucose tolerance as well as insulin secretion. Several tissues are affected, including the vasculature, endocrine pancreas, insulin sensitive tissues, kidney and brain[40].

Some of the pathological changes can develop after a delay and there are intergenerational effects. The effects may cause degenerative diseases in adults and they can occur without major changes in birth weight, suggesting that birth weight on its own may be a poor proxy for intra-uterine events.

Postnatal diet

Epidemiological evidence from the Helsinki study[39] and others, suggest that postnatal diet influences the incidence of adult disease originally programmed by poor nutrition *in utero*. In the rat, manipulation of dietary carbohydrate to protein ratio from weaning until adulthood following low protein *in utero* alters gene expression of hepatic fibrinogen genes[79].

Conclusions

We suggest that extensive animal studies are now needed to uncover the specific mechanisms by which altered fetomaternal nutrition and amino acid metabolism lead to degenerative diseases in the offspring. Only when the perinatal origins of these human diseases are established, will it be possible to devise methods for their primary prevention.

References

1   Barker DJP. *Mothers, Babies and Health in Later Life*, 2nd edn, Churchill Livingstone, Edinburgh 1998

2   Hales CN, Barker DJP. Type 2 (non-insulin dependent) diabetes mellitus: the thrifty phenotype hypothesis. *Diabetologia* 1992; **35**: 595–601

3   Stewart RJ, Preele RF, Sheppart HG. 12 generations of marginal protein deficiency. *Br J Nutr* 1997; **33**: 233–53

4   Winick M, Noble A. Cellular response in rats during malnutrition at various ages. *J Nutr* 1966; **89**: 300–6

5   Weinkove C, Weinkove EA, Pimstone BL. Microassays for glucose and insulin. *S Afr Med J* 1974; **48**: 365–8

6   Swenne I, Crace CJ, Milner RD. Persistent impairment of insulin secretory response to glucose in adult rats after limited period of protein-calorie malnutrition early in life. *Diabetes* 1987; **36**: 454–8

7   Snoeck A, Remacle C, Reusens B *et al*. Effects of low protein diet during pregnancy on the fetal rat endocrine pancreas. *Biol Neonate* 1990; **57**: 107–18

8   Woodall SM, Breier BH, Johnston BM *et al* A model of intrauterine growth retardation caused by chronic maternal undernutrition in the rat: effects on the somatotrophic axis and postnatal growth. *J Endocrinol* 1996; **150**: 231–42

9   Gluckman PD, Cutfield W, Harding JE *et al*. Metabolic consequences of intrauterine growth retardation. *Acta Paediatr* 1996; **417**: 53–6

10 Holemans K, Gerber R, Meurren SK *et al*. Maternal food restriction in the 2nd half of pregnancy affects vascular function but not blood pressure of rat female offspring *Br J Nutr* 1999; **81**: 83–9

11 Kind KL, Clifton PM, Katsman AI *et al*. Restricted fetal growth and the response to dietary cholesterol in the guinea pig. *Am J Physiol* 1999; **277**: R1675–82

12 Waterland RA, Garza C. Potential mechanisms of metabolic imprinting that lead to chronic disease *Am J Clin Nutr* 1999; **69**: 179–97

13 Hawkins P, Steyn C, McGarrigle HH *et al*. Effect of maternal nutrient restriction in early gestation on development of the hypothalamic-pituitary-adrenal axis in fetal sheep at 0.8–0.9 of gestation. *J Endocrinol* 1999; **163**: 553–61

14 Hawkins P, Steyn C, McGarrigle HH *et al*. Effect of maternal nutrient restriction on responses of the hypothalamic-pituitary-adrenal axis to acute isocapnic hypoxaemia in late gestation fetal sheep. *Exp Physiol* 2000; **85**: 85–96

15 Langley-Evans SC. Critical differences between two low protein diet protocols in the programming of hypertension in the rat. *Int J Food Sci Nutr* 2000; **51**: 11–7

16 Hales CN, Desai M, Ozanne SE, Crowther NJ. Fishing in the stream of diabetes: from measuring insulin to the control of fetal organogenesis. *Biochem Soc Trans* 1996; **24**: 341–50

17 Rees WD, Hay SM, Buchan V *et al* The effects of maternal protein restriction on the growth of the rat fetus and its amino acid supply. *Br J Nutr* 1999; **81**: 243–50

18 de Gasparo M, Milner GR, Norris P *et al*. Effect of glucose amino acid on fetal rat pancreatic growth and insulin secretion *in vitro*. *J Endocrinol* 1978; **77**: 241–8

19 Reusens B, Dahri S, Snoeck A *et al*. Long term consequences of diabetes and its complications may have a fetal origin: experimental and epidemiological evidence. In: Cowett RM. (ed) *Nestle Nutrition Workshop Series*, vol 25. *Diabetes*. New York: Raven, 1995; 187–98

20 Kwong WY, Wild AE, Roberts P *et al*. Maternal undernutrition during the preimplantation period of rat development causes blastocyst abnormalities and programming of postnatal hypertension. *Development* 2000; **127**: 4195–202

21 Petrik J, Reusens B, Arany E, Remacle C, Coelho C, Hoet JJ, Hill DJ. A low protein diet alters the balance of islet cell replication and apoptosis in the fetal and neonatal rat and is

associated with a reduced pancreatic expression of IGF II. *Endocrinology* 1999; **140**: 4861–73

22 Dahri S, Cherif H, Reusens B *et al* Effect of an isocaloric low protein diet during gestation in the rat on *in vitro* insulin secretion by islets of the offspring. *Diabetologia* 1994; **37 (Suppl 1)**: A80

23 Hoet JJ, Hanson MA Intrauterine nutrition: its importance during critical periods of cardiovascular and endocrine development. *J Physiol* 1999; **514**: 617–27

24 Resnick O, Morgan PJ. Generational effect of protein malnutrition in the rat. *Dev Brain Res* 1984; **15**: 219–27

25 Ozanne SE, Smith GD, Tikerpae J, Hales CN. Altered regulation of hepatic glucose output in the male offspring of protein-malnourished rat dams. *Am J Physiol* 1996; **270**: E559–64

26 Desai M, Crowther NJ, Ozanne SE, Lucas A, Hales CN. Adult glucose and lipid metabolism may be programmed during fetal life. *Biochem Soc Trans* 1995; **23**: 331–5

27 Shepherd PR, Crowther NJ, Desai M, Hales CN, Ozanne SE. Altered adipocyte properties in the offspring of protein malnourished rats. *Br J Nutr* 1997; **78**: 121–9

28 Ozanne SE, Wang CL, Coleman N *et al*. Altered muscle insulin sensitivity in the male offspring of protein malnourished rats. *Am J Physiol* 1996; **271**: E1128–34

29 Ozanne SE, Nave BT, Wang CL *et al*. Poor fetal nutrition causes a long term change in expression of insulin signalling components in adipocytes. *Am J Physiol* 1997; **273**: E46–51

30 Jones AP, Friedman MI. Obesity and adipocyte abnormalities in offspring of rats undernourished during pregnancy. *Science* 1982; **215**: 1518–9

31 Anguita RM, Sigulem DM, Sawaya AL. Intrauterine food restriction is associated with obesity in young rats. *J Nutr* 1993; **123**: 1421–8

32 Hoet JJ, Reusens B, Bahri S, El-Hajjaji H, Remacle CV, van Velzen D. Protein malnutrition during pregnancy in the rat has an intergeneration effect on the endocrine pancreas. In *16th International Congress of Nutrition, Montreal, Canada*, 1992; 70

33 Dahri S, Snoeck A, Reusens-Billen B *et al*. Islet function in offspring of mothers on low-protein diet during gestation. *Diabetes* 1991; **40**: 115–20

34 McCance DR, Pettitt DJ, Hanson RL *et al*. Birthweight and non-insulin dependent diabetes: thrifty genotype, thrifty phenotype, or surviving small baby genotype. *BMJ* 1994; **308**: 942–5

35 Newman WP, Freedman DS, Voors AW *et al*. Relation of serum lipoprotein levels and systolic blood pressure to early atherosclerosis: the Bogalusa Heart Study. *N Engl J Med* 1986; **314**: 138–44

36 Guo F, Jen KLC. High fat feeding during pregnancy and lactation affects offspring metabolism in rats. *Physiol Behav* 1995; **57**: 681–6

37 Brown SA, Rogers LK, Dunn JK *et al*. Development of cholesterol homeostatic memory in the rat is influenced by maternal diets. *Metab Clin Exp* 1990; **39**: 468–73

38 Langley-Evans SC. Intrauterine programming of hypertension in the rat: nutrient interactions. *Comp Biochem Physiol* 1996; **114**: 327–31

39 Eriksson JG, Forsen T, Tuomilehto B *et al*. Catch-up growth in childhood and death from coronary heart disease: longitudinal study. *BMJ* 1999; **318**: 427–31

40 Gardner DS, Jackson AA, Langley-Evans SC. Maintenance of maternal diet-induced hypertension in the rat is dependent on glucocorticoids. *Hypertension* 1997; **30**: 1525–30

41 Tonkiss J, Trzcinska M, Galler JR *et al*. Prenatal malnutrition induced changes in blood pressure. *Hypertension* 1998; **32**: 108–14

42 Aerts L, Holemans K, van Assche FA. Maternal diabetes during pregnancy: consequences for the offspring. *Diabetes Metab Rev* 1990; **16**: 147–97

43 Holemans K, Aerts L, van Assche FA. Evidence for an insulin resistance in the adult offspring of pregnant STZ diabetic rats. *Diabetologia* 1991; **34**: 80–5

44 Koukkou E, Lowry C, Poston L. The offspring of diabetic rats fed a high saturated fat diet in pregnancy demonstrate vascular dysfunction. *Circulation* 1998; **98**: 2899–904

45 Goland RS, Tropper PJ, Warren WB, Stark RI, Jozac SM, Conwell IM. Concentrations of corticotropin-releasing hormone in the umbilical-cord blood of pregnancies complicated by pre-eclampsia. Reprod Fertil Dev 1995; **7**: 1227–30

46 Bjorntorp P, Holm G, Rosmond R. Hypothalamic arousal, insulin resistance and Type 2 diabetes mellitus. *Diabet Med* 1999; **16**: 373–83

47 Walker BR, Phillips DI, Noon JP *et al*. Increased glucocorticoid activity in men with cardiovascular risk factors. *Hypertension* 1998; **31**: 891–5

48 Phillips DIW, Barker DJ, Fall CH *et al*. Elevated plasma cortisol concentrations: a link between low birthweight and the insulin resistance syndrome? *J Clin Endocrinol Metab* 1998; **83**: 757–60

49 Bertram C, Trowern AR, Copin N, Jackson AA, Whorwood CB. The maternal diet during pregnancy programs altered expression of the glucocorticoid receptor and type IIβ–HSD: potential molecular mechanisms underlying the programming of hypertension *in utero*. *Endocrinology* 2001; **142**: 2841–53

50 Langley-Evans SC, Gardner DS, Jackson AA. Maternal protein restriction influences the programming of the rat hypothalamic-pituitary-adrenal axis. *J Nutr* 1996; **126**: 1578–85

51 Langley-Evans SC. Maternal carbenoxolone treatment lowers birthweight and induces hypertension in offspring of rats fed a protein replete diet *Clin Sci* 1997; **93**: 423–9

52 Bertram C, Trowern AR, Whorwood CB. Maternal low protein treatment but not Carbenoxolone treatment results in persistent upregulation of glucocorticoid receptor in central and peripheral tissues *J Endocrinol* 1999; **163**: P62

53 McMillen IC, Warnes KE, Adams MB *et al*. Impact of restriction of placental and fetal growth on expression of 11β-HSD1 and 2 mRNA in the liver, kidney and adrenal of the sheep fetus. *Endocrinology* 2000; **141**: 539–43

54 Lindsay RS, Lindsay RM, Waddell BJ *et al*. Prenatal glucocorticoid exposure leads to offspring hyperglycaemia in the rat: studies with the 11β-HSD inhibitor carbenoxolone. *Diabetologia* 1996; **39**: 1299–305

55 Nyirenda MJ, Lindsay RS, Kenyon CJ *et al*. Glucocorticoid exposure in late gestation permanently programs rat hepatic PEPCK and GR expression and causes glucose intolerance in adult offspring. *J Clin Invest* 1998; **101**: 2174–81

56 Langley-Evans SC. Intrauterine programming of hypertension by glucocorticoids. *Life Sci* 1997; **60**: 1213–21

58 Dodic M, May CN, Coghlan JP. Carbenoxolone does not cause a syndrome of mineralocorticoid excess in sheep. *Steroids* 1998; **63**: 99–104

59 Benediktsson R, Linsday RS, Noble J, Seckl JR. Glucocorticoid exposure *in utero*: new model for adult hypertension. *Lancet* 1993; **341**: 339–41

60 Gatford KL, Wintour EM, de Blasio MJ *et al* Differential timing for programming of glucose homeostasis, sensitivity to insulin and blood pressure by *in utero* exposure to dexamethasone in sheep. *Clin Sci* 2000; **98**: 553–60

61 McCarty R, Lee JH. Maternal influences in adult blood pressure of SHRs: a single-pup cross-fostering study. *Physiol Behav* 1996; **59**: 71–7

63 Liu JP, Baker J, Perkins AS *et al*. Mice carrying null mutations of the genes encoding IGF1 and IGF1r. *Cell* 1993; **75**: 59–72

64 Petrik J, Pell JM, Arany E *et al* Overexpression of insulin-like growth factor-II in transgenic mice is associated with pancreatic islet cell hyperplasia. *Endocrinology* 1999; **140**: 2353–63

65 Withers DJ, Gutierrez JS, Towery H *et al*. Disruption of IRS-2 causes type 2 diabetes in mice. *Nature* 1998; **391**: 900–4

66 Kulkarni RN, Bruning JC, Winnay JN, Postic C, Magnuson MA, Kahn CR. Tissue-specific knockout of the insulin receptor in pancreatic beta cells creates an insulin secretory defect similar to that in type 2 diabetes. *Cell* 1999; **96**: 329–39

67 Jacobson L. Lower weight loss and food intake in protein deprived, CRH-deficient mice correlate with glucocorticoid insufficiency. *Endocrinology* 1999; **140**: 3543–51

68 Persson E, Jansson T. Low birthweight is associated with elevated adult blood pressure in the chronically catheterised guinea pig. *Acta Physiol Scand* 1992; **145**: 195-6

69 Jansson T, Lambert GW. Effect of intrauterine growth restriction on blood pressure, glucose tolerance and sympathetic nervous system activity in the rat at 3–4 months of age. *J Hypertens* 1999; **17**: 1239–48

70 Harding J. Nutritional causes of impaired fetal growth and their treatment. *J R Soc Med* 1999; **92**: 612–5

71 Murotsuki J, Challis JR, Han VK *et al*. Chronic fetal placental embolism and hypoxaemia cause hypertension and myocardial hypertrophy in fetal sheep. *Am J Physiol* 1997; **272**: R201–7

72 Murotsuki J, Gagnon R, Pu X *et al*. Chronic hypoxaemia selectively down-regulates 11β-HSD2 gene expression in the fetal sheep kidney. *Biol Reprod* 1998; **58**: 234–9

73 Reik W, Murrell A. Genomic imprinting. Silence across the border. *Nature* 2000; **405**: 408–9

74 Harel Z, Tannenbaum GS. Long-term alterations in growth hormone and insulin secretion after temporary dietary protein restriction in the early life of the rat. *Pediatr Res* 1995; **38**: 747–53

75 Hawkins P, Crowe C, Calder NA *et al*. Cardiovascular development in late gestation fetal sheep and young lambs following modest maternal nutrient restriction in early gestation. *J Physiol* 1997; **505**: 18P

76 Hawkins P, Crowe C, McGarrigle HHG *et al*. Effect of maternal nutrient restriction in early gestation on hypothalamic pituitary adrenal axis responses during acute hypoxaemia in late gestation fetal sheep. *J Physiol* 1998; **507**: 50P

77 Edwards CRW, Benediktsson R, Lindsay RS *et al*. Dysfunction of placental glucocorticoid barrier: link between fetal environment and adult hypertension. *Lancet* 1993; **341**: 355–7

78 Norman LJ, Challis J. Synergism between corticotrophin-releasing factor and arginine vasopressin and adrenocorticotrophin release *in vivo* varies as function of gestational age in the ovine fetus. *Endocrinology* 1987; **120**: 1052–8

79 Zhang J, Desai M, Ozanne SE *et al* Two variants of quantitative reverse transcriptase PCR used to show differential expression of fibrinogen genes in rat liver lobes. *Biochem J* 1997; **321**: 769–75

Intra-uterine programming of the endocrine pancreas

Abigail L Fowden* and **David J Hill**[†]

Department of Physiology, University of Cambridge, Cambridge, UK and †Lawson Health Research Institute, University of Western Ontario, Ontario, Canada

In altricial species such as the rat and mouse, there is good evidence for the intra-uterine programming of the endocrine pancreas. Changes in the intra-uterine nutritional environment cause alterations in the structure and function of the islets which have life-long effects and predispose the animal to glucose intolerance and diabetes in later life. In rodents, the islets develop relatively late in gestation and undergo substantial remodelling in the period immediately after birth. Hence, the critical window for islet development in these animals is short and readily accessible for experimental manipulation. The short life-span of these species also means that elderly animals can be studied within a reasonable time frame. In precocious species, such as guinea pigs and farm animals, intra-uterine programming of the endocrine pancreas is less well established. In part, this may be due to difficulties in identifying the critical window for development as islet formation and remodelling begin at an earlier stage of gestation and continue for longer after birth. The long life-span of these animals and the relative insulin resistance of adult ruminants compared to other species also make it difficult to establish whether fetal changes in islet development have long-term consequences. In the human, the main phase of islet development occurs during the second trimester, although remodelling occurs throughout late gestation and early childhood. There is, therefore, a relatively long period in which early changes in islet development could be reversed or ameliorated in the human. Although the human epidemiological observations suggest that the fetal origin of adult glucose intolerance is due primarily to changes in insulin sensitivity rather than to defective insulin secretion, subtle changes in islet morphology and function sustained *in utero* may well contribute to the increased susceptibility to type 2 diabetes observed in adults who were growth-retarded *in utero*.

Correspondence to:
Dr Abigail L Fowden,
Department of
Physiology, University of
Cambridge, Cambridge
CB2 3EG, UK

Human epidemiological studies have shown that impaired growth *in utero* is associated with an increased incidence of glucose intolerance and type 2 diabetes in later life and linked this to poor nutrition during pregnancy and/or early infancy. In part, the changes in glucose tolerance observed in the elderly human populations may be due to alterations in

---

pancreatic endocrine function sustained *in utero*. The evidence for the intra-uterine programming of islet function is discussed in this chapter.

Normal development of the endocrine pancreas

Morphogenesis

Morphogenesis of the endocrine pancreas appears to follow a similar sequence in all mammals although the precise stage of gestation at which the specific events occur may vary amongst species[1]. The pancreas develops from two diverticula of the primitive gut which fuse during early embryonic growth to form both the exocrine and endocrine pancreas. The endocrine tissue is derived from epithelial duct cells by rotation of the plane of mitotic division. (Fig. 1). The single immature endocrine cells derived from the duct epithelia multiply and form small knots of cells which bud out of the pancreatic ducts (Fig. 1). In humans, this process of budding is observed as early as 10 weeks of gestation[2,3]. The clusters of immature endocrine cells become vascularized by 16 weeks of gestation in humans and are then encapsulated by connective

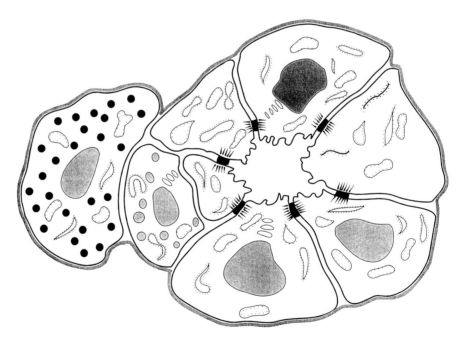

Fig. 1 Schematic diagram of the formation of endocrine cells in the fetal pancreas. Duct cells dividing parallel to the lumen undergo endocrine differentiation and bud off from the duct cell to form immature, undifferentiated endocrine cells (stippled granules) which proliferate and differentiate into mature endocrine cells (solid granules).

tissue and isolated from the ducts[2,3]. At this stage of development, the endocrine cells are still relatively undifferentiated and the cytoplasmic granules co-localize several pancreatic hormones and neuropeptides[4]. During the second half of gestation, the developing islets become innervated and the individual cell types differentiate to contain only a single pancreatic hormone[5,6]. The numbers and spatial arrangement of the 4 different endocrine cell types within the islets, therefore, change during the third trimester but, by term, some of the islets have the appearance and topography characteristic of mature adult islets of Langerhans[3]. In total, the islets account for about 4% of the total pancreas in the normal human infant at birth.

Further re-organization of the pancreatic endocrine tissue occurs after birth, with changes in islet size and topography in most species[1,3,5]. The duration of this postnatal period of islet remodelling depends on species and varies from 4 weeks in the rat to 4 years or more in the human infant[3,5]. In the rat, the main phase of remodelling occurs around weaning at 2–3 weeks of postnatal age and is associated with a wave of islet cell apoptosis[7]. The mass of endocrine tissue in the neonatal pancreas, therefore, depends on three processes: (i) neogenesis from the duct epithelia; (ii) proliferation of the cells committed to endocrine differentiation; and (iii) apoptosis of the endocrine cells to remodel the developing islets.

Functional development

The pancreatic hormones can be extracted from the fetal pancreas before the various cell types can be distinguished readily[1,8]. For most of gestation, the glucagon containing α cells predominate and are the first cell type to be identified clearly, mainly in the periphery of the pancreas during early embryonic development[3,8]. In most species, α-cells appear before β-cells with δ- and PP cells becoming detectable later in gestation[8]. By birth, the ratio of α- to β-cells has decreased and closely resembles that seen in adults, at least in humans. The pancreatic content of insulin and glucagon increases with increasing gestational age in parallel with the increase in cell number in several species including the human[5,8,9].

The synthesis and release of the pancreatic hormones in the fetus appears to occur in a manner similar to that observed in the adult[10]. In the β-cells, all the key elements involved in stimulus–secretion coupling in the adult have been identified in the fetus. Insulin secretion occurs by exocytosis of the granules into the intercellular space, where the insulin storage complex breaks down. Pulse chase and immunohistochemical analysis show that prohormones are formed and stored in the granules of the fetal islet cells[11]. Conversion of pro-insulin to insulin appears to

Table 1 The gestational age at which insulin and glucagon are first detected in the fetal pancreas and plasma in different species

Species	Length of gestation (days)	Insulin		Glucagon	
		Pancreas (days)	Plasma (days)	Pancreas (days)	Plasma (days)
Rat	23	12	18	11	18
Sheep	147	40	60	40	60
Human	280	70	84	42	77

occur in the granules as very little pro-insulin is detected in the fetal circulation. Paracrine interactions between the different endocrine cells in the islet also occur in the fetus as selective ablation of the β-cells leads to an increase in plasma glucagon in the sheep fetus[10,12].

Insulin and glucagon can be measured in fetal plasma shortly after they are detected in the pancreas (Table 1), while somatostatin and pancreatic polypeptide are present in fetal plasma by term[10]. The actual concentrations of the pancreatic hormones in the fetal circulation vary widely amongst species and also change with gestational age. For instance, in late gestation, fetal plasma insulin is 200 μU/ml in the rat but only 10 μU/ml in the pig and horse[10,13]. In the majority of species, including the human, insulin and glucagon concentrations rise between mid and late gestation and then remain stable until near term.

The fetal α- and β-cells are sensitive to secretogogues *in utero*[10]. Changes in fetal insulin and glucagon secretion have been observed in response to a range of stimuli including metabolites, neurotransmitters and hormones[10]. The fetal β-cell responses to glucose and amino acids show developmental changes with increasing gestational age in both *in vivo* and *in vitro* studies[14–16]. During late gestation, the fetal β-cells respond readily to changes in the glucose and amino acid levels and are also affected by circulating catecholamine levels and adverse conditions such as hypoxia and anaesthesia. In contrast, fetal α-cells appear to be relatively unresponsive to changes in the glucose level, unlike neonatal or adult α-cells[10]. However, fetal α-cells respond rapidly to changes in the level of amino acids and catecholamines which suggest that it is the glucose sensing mechanisms rather than the synthesis and release of glucagon that may be immature in fetal α-cells. In addition, the autonomic nerves to the fetal pancreas are active by late gestation and involved in regulating islet cell responses to stressful stimuli.

Glucose has been shown to stimulate insulin secretion both in the fetus *in utero* and in *in vitro* experiments with cultured islet cells in several species[10,13,14,17]. The initial *in vitro* studies also showed that the fetal β-cell response to glucose was slow and of smaller magnitude than those seen in cultured new-born or adult islet cells[1,10,13]. Since the fetal β-cell responses to amino acids and other secretogogues were similar to those of adult cells *in vitro*, the poor response to glucose was attributed to immaturity of the glucose sensing mechanisms in the fetal β-cells[1,13]. However, β-cell function may have been adversely affected in the *in vitro* studies by the isolation of the islet cells. In unstressed, chronically catheterised fetuses, the β-cell response to exogenous glucose is relatively rapid with a significant rise in plasma insulin within 5-10 min of raising the fetal glucose concentration[10]. With prolonged glucose infusion, the fetal insulin levels continue to rise to a plateau value, but do not show the rapid early phase of the typical biphasic response observed postnatally[10,14]. However, since fetal β-cells would not normally experience sudden or large changes in the glucose level of the type observed during exogenous glucose administration, the apparent immaturity of glucose-stimulated insulin release *in utero* is not physiologically relevant. Indeed, fetal insulin levels are positively correlated with the glucose level over the range of values normally observed *in utero* in several species[10]. Fetal β-cells, therefore, show appropriate responses to the changes in glucose levels that occur *in utero* and have a physiological role in regulating fetal metabolism.

The fetal α- and β-cells have important roles in fetal growth and development[11]. Insulin secretion from the β-cells is essential for glucose uptake by the insulin-sensitive tissues of the fetus. Ablation of the fetal β-cells leads to hyperglycaemia, reduced glucose utilization and, ultimately, growth retardation of the fetus. The fetal β-cells, therefore, act as sensors of nutrient sufficiency and, via insulin secretion, match the rates of glucose utilization and growth by the fetus to its rate of glucose supply. On the other hand, fetal α-cells appears to act as sensors of nutrient insufficiency, particularly of oxygen. Glucagon raises fetal glucose levels and has effects on the fetal cardiovascular system at high concentrations. These changes may help maintain a glucose supply to essential fetal tissues, such as the brain during adverse intra-uterine conditions[11].

Factors affecting development of the endocrine pancreas *in utero*

In the human infant, the percentage of islet tissue in the pancreas at birth is positively correlated to birth weight[1,11]. In growth retarded and small-for-date infants, the percentage of islet tissue is reduced from 4% to only 2% of the total pancreas. Basal and glucose-stimulated levels of insulin are also low in these infants[5,11]. These clinical observations suggest that adverse intra-uterine conditions which lower birth weight also impair development of the fetal endocrine pancreas. In experimental animals, islet development has been shown to be affected by various transcription factors and by the intra-uterine availability of specific metabolites, hormones and growth factors[5,13,17,18]. These variables alter both the structural and functional development of the endocrine pancreas, although their specific effects depends on the severity, duration and gestational age at onset of the perturbation.

Transcription factors

The development of ductal epithelial cells into an endocrine lineage, and ultimately into β-cells, involves a specific sequence of expression of transcription factors[19]. One of the most important identified so far is Pdx-1, also known as STF-1, IDX-1 or IPF-1[20]. In animals with a targeted deletion of *Pdx*-1, pancreatic buds form but no further differentiation or morphogenesis occurs[21]. However, some β-cells are found in the pancreatic rudiments, showing that Pdx-1 is not obligatory for β-cell differentiation and insulin secretion. Expression of *Pdx*-1 in undifferentiated ductal epithelium is associated with the glucose transporter GLUT 2, which by day 15 of gestation in the fetal rat has been lost from acinar cells, but is retained by developing β-cells. Pdx-1, therefore, appears to have a dual role, in the induction of an early endocrine cell lineage from ductal epithelial cells, and in the maturation of β-cells and insulin gene expression. A single deletion of a nucleotide in the human *Pdx*-1 gene leads to complete pancreatic agenesis[22]. Thus, control of Pdx-1 expression may be a key step in pancreatic development. Pdx-1 expression is directed by at least two other nuclear transcription factors, hepatocyte nuclear factor 3β (HNF-3β) and BETA-2/NeuroD.

Neogenesis of β-cells is also affected by members of the Pax gene family. Pax-4 and Pax-6 are expressed in the developing pancreas and deletion of *Pax*-4 in mouse has been shown to cause a complete loss of pancreatic β-cells and δ-cells, but an increased number of α-cells[23]. Conversely, functional deletion of the *Pax*-6 gene in the mouse decreases the presence of all four endocrine cell types in the pancreas, with the presence of α-cells being totally abolished[24]. Pax-6 has been shown to *trans*-activate both the glucagon and insulin gene promoters. Mice lacking both Pax-4 and Pax-6 failed to develop any mature endocrine cells in the pancreas. Pax-4 and Pax-6, therefore, appear to be important at a later stage of development than Pdx-1, distinguishing the α-cell lineage from the β- and δ-cell lines.

Genetic lesions within transcription factors governing pancreatic development have been found to underlie some forms of diabetes. Maturity-onset diabetes of the young (MODY), a form of type-2 diabetes, is a monogenic disease with autosomal dominant inheritance, and is characterized by an early onset of failure of insulin secretion[25]. The known genes that are involved in MODY are hepatocyte nuclear factor 4α (*HNF-4α*) (MODY 1)[26], glucokinase (MODY 2)[27,28], *HNF-1α* (MODY 3)[29], and *Pdx-1* (MODY 4)[30]. MODY 4 has been observed in patients carrying a heterozygous mutation in *Pdx-1*. The resulting phenotype differed widely between individuals, some being normal others being glucose intolerant, suggesting that penetrance of this mutation was not complete. The expression of the HNF factors were first found in the liver, but a role in the pancreas now also seems likely, as, in MODY 3, there is an impaired insulin secretion[31]. A family of patients with MODY1 has been described with mutations in *HNF-4α* who developed diabetes requiring insulin therapy in 30% of cases[26]. Such patients demonstrate primary defects in the mechanisms releasing insulin in the β-cells[32,33].

Availability of nutrients

Development of fetal islet cells have been shown to be dependent on the availability of glucose and amino acids in both *in vivo* and *in vitro* studies[5,10,13,14,15,34]. Cultured islet cells from fetal rats require both glucose and amino acids for normal development[35]. At 17–18 days of gestation, amino acids appear to be more important than glucose whereas, by term, glucose has become the critical factor in islet development *in vitro*[1,5,13]. Similarly, in mice, glucose availability to the islet cells has a more pronounced effect on their development postnatally than prenatally[36]. This developmental shift in nutrient dependence is consistent with the changes in nutrition that occur at birth. Prenatally, amino acid levels are high and glucose levels are low, whereas postnatally glucose is more plentiful than amino acids.

In vivo, islet development is altered by both decreases and increases in nutrient availability. In rats, maternal metabolic perturbations induced by diabetes or reductions in dietary intake of protein or calories during pregnancy alter development of the β-cells in the fetal islets[5,13,18,37–39]. Feeding a low protein (LP) isocalorific diet (8% protein) to pregnant rats changes amino acid profiles but has little, if any, effect on glycaemia in the fetus and mother[13]. In late gestation, the fetal islets from LP rats were smaller and contained less β-cells and insulin than those from control animals fed a normal diet (20% protein) during pregnancy[18,38]. Protein deprivation during pregnancy, therefore, alters the balance between neogenesis, proliferation and apoptosis in the fetal islets[40]. Proliferation of the existing islet cells was reduced while apoptosis was increased in the fetal islets of LP rats[40]. The cell cycle of the fetal islet cells was also lengthened in these circumstances[40]. The fetal islets from the LP animals were also poorly vascularized and released less insulin in response to secretogogues such as glucose and amino acids[38,41]. The reductions in islet cell proliferation and amino acid stimulated insulin release were maintained when fetal islets from LP rats were cultured for 7 days[13,42]. Protein deprivation *in utero*, therefore, induces permanent changes in the growth and function of the fetal islet cells.

Reduction in total calorific intake during pregnancy also affects development of the fetal endocrine pancreas but in a different manner to that seen with protein deprivation. Like protein deprivation, reducing calorific intake by 50% for the last 7 days of pregnancy in rats leads to decreases in β-cell mass and insulin content of the fetal pancreas[13,42]. However, this reduction in β-cell mass appears to be due to reduced neogenesis and a smaller number of islets rather than to lower rates of β-cell proliferation as occurs with protein deprivation[42]. In pregnant sheep, prolonged maternal hypoglycaemia induced by insulin infusion leads to a reduced fetal insulin level and a decrease in glucose-stimulated insulin release[14]. Restricting nutrient availability either in total or of glucose, in particular, therefore reduces fetal β-cell mass and increases the α- to β-cell ratio in the fetal islets during development.

Raising fetal glucose levels by maternal diabetes induces changes in islet development which are determined by the severity of the diabetes (*see also* Van Assche *et al*, this issue). Moderate maternal diabetes in rats leads to an increase in the fetal pancreatic insulin content, enhanced insulin secretion in response to glucose and greater proliferation of the islet cells[13,35]. Similar increases in insulin secretion are seen in sheep fetuses in which maternal glucose levels were raised periodically by pulsatile glucose infusion[15]. On the other hand, severe diabetes or maintained experimental maternal hyperglycaemia leads to a decrease in the insulin content and degranulation of the β-cells in fetal sheep and rats[12,34,35]. These fetuses also have low circulating insulin levels and a reduced β-cell response to exogenous glucose. A reduced β-cell mass and degranulation of the β-cells has also been observed in an infant of a severely diabetic women[1]. These observations suggest that severe, prolonged hyperglycaemia *in utero* has adverse effects on pancreatic endocrine development and leads to β-cell exhaustion.

Glucose availability, therefore, appears to have an important role in islet development *in vivo*. However, since maternal amino acid levels are also altered by maternal diabetes, calorific restriction and experimental hypoglycaemia, some of the apparent effects of variations in glycaemia may be due, in part, to changes in amino acid profile. Certainly, for most of gestation, amino acids appear to be more important than glucose in stimulating β-cell proliferation *in vitro*[13,42]. In addition, replacement of a single amino acid, taurine, in the drinking water of pregnant rats fed 8% protein prevented the reduction in β-cell mass and pancreatic insulin content in the fetuses in late gestation[37]. Some of the changes in islet development may be due to the nutritionally-induced alterations in exposure to hormones and growth factors[43]. For instance, maternal protein deprivation reduces placental 11β hydroxysteroid dehydrogenase activity which, in turn, increases fetal exposure to maternal glucocorticoids[44].

Availability of hormones and growth factors

Pancreatic islet development has been shown to be influenced by a number of growth factors including the protein complex, ilotrophin, the fibroblast growth factor (FGF) family, platelet derived growth factor, transforming growth factor-α (TGF-α) and the insulin-like growth factors, IGF-I and IGF-II[45]. Islet neogenesis associated protein (INGAP), part of the ilotrophin complex, is believed to initiate duct cell proliferation and endocrine cell differentiation. INGAP, TGF-α and platelet derived growth factor have all been identified in the fetal pancreas, but little is known about their ontogeny or control during islet development[19,45]. Much more is known about the IGFs and FGFs.

Exogenous FGF-1 was able to increase the insulin content of fetal rat 'islet-like structures'[46] which suggests that it may potentiate β-cell generation. However, FGF-7 may be a more potent inducer of β-cell neogenesis. Systemic injection of FGF-7 into adult rats for up to 2 weeks caused a rapid increase in DNA synthesis within the ductal epithelium which was seen within 24 h[47]. Pancreatic duct hyperplasia followed, but not a progression to increased numbers of endocrine cells. When FGF-7 was expressed within the embryonic liver of transgenic mice, driven by an ApoE promoter, pancreatic duct hyperplasia was seen, with increased numbers of ductal cells containing immunoreactive insulin[48]. The ability of circulating FGF-7 to promote β-cell neogenesis in the embryo, but only cause ductal cell proliferation in the adult, suggests that additional growth factors are necessary to complete the neogenic process *in utero*. In neonatal rats, FGF-7 immunoreactivity is predominantly associated with stroma around the vascular endothelium of capillaries and ducts[49]. This is consistent with its reported origins within mesenchymal tissues of other organs during embryogenesis, while target cells expressing the FGF-4 receptor are located within adjacent epithelia[50].

The fetal pancreas expresses IGF-I, IGF-II and IGF binding protein 3 during late gestation[51]. As in other fetal tissues, IGF-II is the predominant IGF in the pancreas and is localised to the islets and duct epithelial cells[45,52]. Both IGF-I and IGF-II are mitogens in the fetal pancreas and lead to an increase in islet cell mass[51]. Transgenic IGF-II mice which over-express IGF-II *in utero* are larger at birth and show abnormalities in pancreatic endocrine development[53]. The fetal islets are irregular in shape and 5 times greater in area than in controls. The islets of fetuses expressing the transgene also had a higher α- to β-cell ratio and altered topography of the endocrine cell types within the islet. In addition, the number of fetal islet cells proliferating increased from the normal value of 11% to 20% in those with high IGF-II levels. There was also decreased apoptosis in the fetal islets of the transgenic animals[53].

Neonatally, pancreatic IGF-II gene expression declines in parallel with the major wave of developmental apoptosis[40]. When circulating IGF-II levels are maintained in mice after birth by transgenic expression of IGF-II by specific non-pancreatic tissues, the wave of apoptosis in the islets is prevented[7]. The islets from the neonates with raised IGF-II levels were larger and had a higher proliferation rate than the wild-type controls. IGF-II has also been shown to increase islet cell survival in neonatal rats exposed to cytokines which normally induce cell death[45]. IGF-II, therefore, appears to be cytoprotective and prevents the developmental apoptosis normally associated with β-cell turnover in neonatal life. Its actions appear to be both paracrine and endocrine and, by altering the balance between proliferation and apoptosis, it has a major influence on the β-cell mass of the developing pancreas.

Expression of the IGFs *in utero* is regulated by a number of factors including nutrient and hormone concentrations[11,45]. *In vitro*, release of IGF-I and IGF-II by cultured fetal rat islets is stimulated by glucose and amino acids[51]. *In vivo*, fetal undernutrition induced by maternal dietary restriction or placental insufficiency reduces expression of both IGF genes in a variety of fetal tissues[42–44]. In rats fed a LP diet during pregnancy, gene expression for IGF-II but not IGF-I was reduced by 40% in the fetal pancreas during late gestation[40]. In addition, increased fetal glucocorticoid exposure has been used to suppress IGF-II and IGF-I gene expression in a developmental and tissue specific manner, although little is known about the effects of natural or synthetic glucocorticoids on pancreatic IGF gene expression[43]. Insulin itself is also believed to regulate fetal IGF production. In fetal sheep, insulin raises IGF-I levels while conversely IGF-I suppresses insulin concentrations[43]. There may, therefore, be intra-islet feedback regulation of insulin and IGF-I secretion which maintains the circulating insulin levels while stimulating an increase in insulin synthesis and β-cell mass during late gestation.

In many fetal tissues, glucocorticoids have an important role in regulating cell proliferation and differentiation, especially during the prepartum period when fetal tissues are maturing in preparation for extra-uterine life[43]. In part, these maturational effects of the glucocorticoids are mediated through changes in IGF gene expression and/or thyroid hormone status. However, little is known about the effects of the glucocorticoids or thyroid hormones on the structural development of the fetal endocrine pancreas. Manipulation of the fetal hypothalamic-pituitary-adrenal or thyroid axes appears to have little effect on basal or glucose stimulated insulin levels in fetal sheep[10]. In contrast, removal of the pituitary hormones by fetal decapitation or hypophysectomy increases fetal insulin levels and enhances insulin secretion in response to glucose in fetal rabbits and pigs[1,10]. A functional hypothalamic pituitary link is also essential for the proliferation of fetal β-cells in the infant of the moderately diabetic women[1]. However, changes in pancreatic innervation in the absence of cerebral tissue may also contribute to the abnormalities in pancreatic endocrine function observed after fetal decapitation and in human anencephalics.

Long-term consequences

Intra-uterine changes in pancreatic endocrine development have long-term consequences for islet function and the regulation of glycaemia in the postnatal animal. The specific effects that abnormalities in fetal islet development have postnatally depend, in part, on the nutritional and hormonal environment experienced after birth. For instance, the poor vascularization of the fetal islets in LP rats is maintained at 3 months of postnatal age if protein restriction continues during lactation, but is ameliorated if the LP neonates are fostered at birth onto rats fed normally during pregnancy and lactation[54]. On the other hand, the pancreatic insulin content is low at 3 months of postnatal age in animals, protein deprived *in utero*, irrespective of whether they were suckling by LP or normally fed rats during lactation[13,42]. Abnormalities in islet development sustained *in utero* can also be unmasked by conditions, such as pregnancy, ageing and obesity, which increase the demand for insulin.

Juvenile animals

At 3 months of age, rats exposed solely to low protein *in utero* still have abnormalities in the structure and function of the endocrine pancreas. Although the vascularity of the islets appeared to be restored to normal, the islets were bigger and contained less insulin than controls[41,54]. *In vitro*, the islets from the 3-month-old rats, protein deprived *in utero*, were less responsive to amino acids but responded normally to glucose[17,18,38,43]. However, *in vivo*, these rats had lower insulin concentrations after an oral glucose load in the female, but not the male animals[38]. The LP females also had higher basal glucagon concentrations at 3 months of age[55]. These observations indicate that male but not female animals are able to recuperate from protein deprivation *in utero* when given a normal diet after birth. They also suggest that the prenatal programming of postnatal islet function may be sex linked and related to differences in exposure to sex steroids *in utero*.

When protein deprivation was maintained during pregnancy and lactation, the changes in the islets of the 3-month-old rats were more extensive[5,13,38,39]. In addition to larger islets and a reduced insulin content[13,38], the pancreas had fewer blood vessels per unit volume and a lower blood flow[54]. The insulin response to amino acids and glucose was also reduced both *in vitro* and *in vivo* in males and females[42]. Similarly, offspring of mothers with restricted calorie intake during pregnancy and lactation had fewer β-cells and secreted less insulin in response to oral glucose administration at 3 months of age[56]. However, with intra-uterine calorie restriction, it appeared to be the males rather than the females that were adversely affected[13,42]. In contrast, offspring of diabetic mothers appear to have a morphologically normal pancreas and normal con-centrations of insulin and glucose at 3 months of age under basal conditions[55]. However, insulin levels were raised in these animals in response to glucose administration *in vivo*. The abnormalities in islet development sustained *in utero* were, therefore, maintained to a greater or lesser extent in all three experimental models (low protein, low calorie, diabetes) used to investigate the intra-uterine programming of the islet function. However, the changes in insulin secretion were rarely associated with alterations in glucose tolerance at 3 months of age because of compensatory changes in insulin sensitivity of the peripheral tissues[39,55,56].

Pregnancy

During normal pregnancy, there is increased β-cell proliferation, enhanced insulin synthesis and a lower threshold for glucose-stimulated insulin secretion[13]. In females, protein deprived either solely *in utero* or during pregnancy and lactation, β-cell proliferation is reduced during pregnancy and the islet cell mass and pancreatic insulin content are low at the end of gestation compared with controls. In some, but not all studies, the insulin response to oral glucose was also smaller than normal in pregnant rats protein deprived in early life[13]. Reduced β-cell proliferation was also observed during pregnancy in the female offspring of rats deprived of calories during pregnancy[42]. In female rats, deprivation of either protein or calories during fetal and early postnatal life therefore leads to gestational diabetes with lower insulin and higher glucose levels than during normal pregnancy. Gestational diabetes also occurs in the female offspring of diabetic rats[35].

Ageing

In contrast to juvenile animals, glucose intolerance is common in elderly rats (11–15 months) which have been deprived of protein or calories or treated with dexamethasone during early life[13,17,43,55,58]. However, in the majority of these studies, the glucose intolerance was the result of insulin resistance rather than defective insulin secretion[39,55,58]. Insulopenia was observed only in the rats deprived of calories pre- and postnatally and in females, but not males, protein restricted during early life. Nutritional manipulations *in utero* may, therefore, accelerate the ageing process so that, by 11–15 months, there is less difference in islet function between control and manipulated animals than seen at 3 months.

In the human population, glucose intolerance is also more frequent in adults older than 50 years who were either small at birth or were calorie deprived during mid to late gestation. Like the animal studies, glucose intolerance in the older human population appeared to be more closely related to insulin insensitivity than insulopenia. However, the basal and glucose-stimulated levels of pro-insulin and 32-33 split pro-insulin were elevated in elderly men who were small at birth or calorie deprived *in utero*[17]. The prohormone convertases in the insulin granules may, therefore, be adversely affected by the intra-uterine environment but only lead to abnormalities in pro-insulin cleavage later in life.

Transgenerational effects

The gestational diabetes that occurs in female offspring (second generation) of rats exposed to metabolic abnormalities during pregnancy in the first generation leads to fetal hyperglycaemia and hypoinsulinaemia in the fetuses in late gestation (third generation). There are also reductions in the volume density of the β-cells and pancreatic insulin content as well as changes in islet size distribution in the fetuses of this third generation[42]. Adults of the third generation, particularly the females, are glucose intolerant and develop type 2 diabetes and its complications in later life[13]. Overall, it takes at least three generations to reverse the effects of moderate malnutrition during pregnancy. However, normalization of glycaemia in the first generation, stretozotocin-induced, diabetic rats by islet cell transplants prevents these transgenerational effects[13,35].

Mechanisms of programming pancreatic endocrine function

There are a wide range of structural and functional changes that can occur in the endocrine pancreas during fetal development that could lead to changes in islet function in later life (Table 2). The changes in the vascularity and vascular reactivity in the islets that occur in response to early protein deprivation may be due to alterations in both locally

Table 2 Processes within the pancreatic β-cell that may be programmed *in utero*

Vascularity of the islets	Number of vessels
	Reactivity of vessels
Innervation of the islets	Number of nerves
	Activity of nerves
	Neurotransmitter release and turnover
Islet morphology	Size of islets within the pancreas
	Number of endocrine cells
	Ratio of endocrine cell types
	Topography of endocrine cell types
Hormone synthesis	Intracellular signalling mechanisms
	Gene expression
	Hormone packaging
	Prohormone convertases (*see* Fig. 2)
Stimulus-secretion coupling (*see* Fig. 2)	Metabolite sensing mechanisms
	Depolarisation
	Ca^{2+} entry
	Exocytosis

produced and blood-borne growth factors such as FGF, VEGF and IGFs[41,45,54]. The endothelium of the islet capillaries expresses a unique nitric oxide (NO) synthetase which is regulated by the glucose concentration[54]. Since NO production in other vascular beds appears to be programmed *in utero*[42], the low blood flow of the adult pancreas of offspring protein deprived in early life may be due to diminished endothelial NO activity in the islets. The low vessel density and blood flow to the pancreas will reduce exposure of the islets to metabolic stimuli and blood-borne growth factors which may limit insulin secretion and postnatal β-cell proliferation with long term consequences for adult β-cell function.

Changes in the pancreatic innervation induced *in utero* may also contribute to the changes in adult islet function. In other tissues, the number of nerve fibres and the activity of these nerves are determined by the nutritional and hormonal environment *in utero*[44]. Circulating catecholamine concentrations are also known to be higher in growth-retarded fetuses than in those normally grown[10]. Furthermore, there is evidence for increased sympathetic activity in adult men who were small at birth. Certainly, the observation that insulin release is suppressed *in vivo* but not *in vitro* in juvenile rats which were protein deprived *in utero*[13,42] suggests that changes in pancreatic innervation or circulating catecholamine levels may be important in regulating insulin secretion *in vivo*.

The changes in islet morphology induced by nutritional manipulation *in utero* have been well documented. In particular, the changes in topography and the α- to β-cell ratio in the islets will affect the local intra-islet regulatory mechanisms and, thereby, alter islet cell responsiveness to physiological stimuli both *in utero* and subsequently. However, the relative contribution of neogenesis, proliferation and apoptosis to the overall changes in islet cell mass and morphology remain unknown and probably differ with the severity, duration and specific nature of the nutritional deficit. Environmental programming may act prior to the generation of endocrine pancreatic cells, at the level of pre-endocrine stem cells within the pancreatic ducts or islets, or even before pancreas formation in the embryo. Using stem cell markers commonly found in preneuronal lineages, such as the intermediary filament protein, nestin, putative pre-endocrine stem cells have been identified both in the pancreatic ducts and within the islets, where they persist in low numbers into adult life[59]. When juvenile rat pancreatic ducts were isolated and allowed to grow as cystic structures *in vitro*, nestin mRNA was detected by RT-PCR after 10 days in culture, before the appearance of insulin-expressing cells. Feeding a low protein diet to pregnant rats significantly reduces the proportion of nestin-expressing stem cells both in the pancreatic ducts and islets of the neonates which suggests a possible environmental limitation of stem cell number and, hence, tissue plasticity in later life.

Much less is known about the intra-uterine programming of the cellular mechanisms controlling the synthesis and release of islet hormones. In the β-cells, activation of insulin synthesis is cAMP dependent. Fetal islets from rat protein deprived during pregnancy release less insulin in response to theophylline and produce less cAMP in response to glucose than controls[13,38]. Together, these findings suggest that there may be nutritionally-induced changes in the adenyl cyclase system which limits insulin synthesis and, ultimately, reduces the insulin response to glucose. The insulin gene contains multiple transcriptional elements that respond to glucose and no single mutation of the rat insulin promotor removes glucose sensitivity[60]. Nutritional and hormonally induced changes in promotor usage *in utero* may alter the translatability of insulin mRNA with consequences for adult insulin secretion. Developmental changes in promotor usage are known to occur with other genes *in utero* and have been shown to be hormone-dependent[44]. In humans, allelic variations in the insulin promotor leads to different insulin genotypes which have been related to birth weight and adult insulin resistance and type 2 diabetes[61]. However, recent studies have indicated that differences in insulin genotype are unlikely to account for much of the association between low birth weight and adult abnormalities in the insulin–glucose relationship[62]. The changes in circulating pro-insulin and 32-33 split pro-insulin seen in elderly human populations that were small at birth or undernourished *in utero* suggests that the final stages of insulin synthesis may be affected by intra-uterine conditions. In particular, the activity of prohormone convertase 2

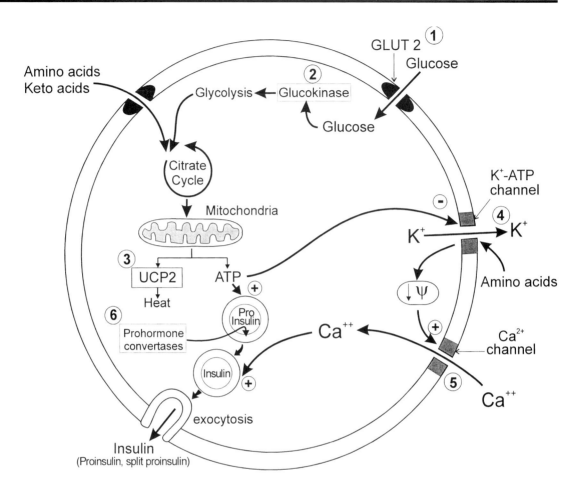

Fig. 2 Diagram of stimulus-secretion coupling in the pancreatic β-cell illustrating the processes which may be programmed *in utero*. 1. Abundance of the glucose transporter-GLUT 2. 2. Abundance and activity of glucokinase. 3. Abundance and activity of uncoupling protein (UCP)-2. 4. ATP-dependent K^+ channels responsible for the potential difference (Ψ) across the cell membrane. 5. Voltage sensitive Ca^{2+} channels responsible for Ca^{2+} entry and $[Ca^{2+}]_i$. 6. Abundance and activity of prohormone convertases which metabolise pro-insulin to insulin.

(PC2) may be reduced in these circumstances (Fig. 2). Neonatal concentrations of 32-33 split pro-insulin are known to be related to maternal intake of energy and protein during pregnancy[16] which indicates that PC2 activity may be nutritionally regulated *in utero*. However, the factors regulating PC activity *in utero* and the extent to which intra-uterine changes in this enzyme activity persist after birth remain unknown.

Finally, stimulus–secretion coupling in the pancreatic endocrine cells may be permanently altered by the intra-uterine environment. There are at least 5 points at which glucose stimulated insulin secretion could be programmed *in utero* (Fig. 2). Glucose is taken up into the β-cell via the GLUT 2 transporter and is then metabolised by glucokinase before entering the citric acid cycle (Fig. 2). GLUT 2 and glucokinase have been identified in the fetal islets from early in gestation in rats and humans[19,36,63]. In human fetal islets, inhibition of GLUT 2 activity reduces insulin release[36]. However, in mice, knockout of GLUT 2 has no effect on the fetal islets which suggests that other glucose transporters may be active *in utero* in this species[63]. In contrast, disruption of the pancreatic glucokinase gene leads to hypoinsulinaemia and growth retardation at birth in both mice and humans[36,64]. Pancreatic gluco-kinase, therefore, appears to be active as a glucose sensor *in utero* and involved in insulin secretion. Total pancreatic glucokinase activity is reduced in 3-month-old rats deprived in early life[65], but little is known about the nutritional or hormonal influences on pancreatic glucokinase and GLUT 2 before birth[66].

Glucose metabolism by the β-cell leads to ATP production which, in turn, closes the ATP-dependent K^+ channel (Fig. 2). Depolarisation of the β-cell results and leads to opening of the voltage-sensitive Ca^{2+} channels. The consequent rise in intracellular Ca^{2+} concentration activates exocytosis and the final release of insulin (Fig. 2). Production of ATP via the citric acid cycle depends, in part, on mitochondrial UCP2 abundance. Disruption of the UCP2 gene in mice leads to hyper-insulinaemia and increases sensitivity to glucose (Lowell B, personal communication). In other fetal tissues, such as brown fat and skeletal muscle, UCP is developmentally regulated and responsive to changes in the availability of nutrients and hormones in the fetus[44]. Patch clamping of the K^+ and Ca^{2+} channels in fetal β-cells showed that their characteristics were similar to those in adults and that the immaturity of glucose-stimulated insulin response in cultured fetal β- cells was upstream of these ion channels[67–69]. Developmental and hormonally induced changes in abundance of K^+ and Ca^{2+} channels have been observed in several fetal and adult tissues[68,69], but nothing is known about the control of these channels in the pancreatic β-cells. Manipulation of pancreatic UCP2 and/or ion channel abundances during intra-uterine growth could, therefore, provide a mechanism of permanently altering β-cell sensitivity to glucose and other secretogogues (Fig. 2).

References

1 Van Assche FA, Aerts L. The fetal endocrine pancreas. *Contrib Gynecol Obstet* 1979; 5: 44–57
2 Bonwens L, Lu WG, De Krijgar RR. Proliferation and differentiation in the human fetal endocrine pancreas. *Diabetologia* 1997; 40: 398–404
3 Robb P. The development of the islets of Langerhans in the human foetus. *Quart J Exp Physiol* 1961; 46: 335–43

4   De Krijgar RR, Aanstoot HJ, Kranenburg G, Reishard M, Visser WJ, Bruining GJ. The mid gestational human fetal pancreas contains cells coexpressing islet hormones. *Dev Biol* 1992; **153**: 368–75

5   Hellerstrom L, Swenne I. Functional maturation and proliferation of fetal pancreatic beta cells. *Diabetes* 1991; **40 (Suppl 2)**: 89–93

6   Portela-Gomes GM, Johansson H, Olding L, Grimelius L. Co-localization of neuroendocrine hormones in the human fetal pancreas. *Eur J Endocrinol* 1999; **141**: 526–33

7   Hill DJ, Strutt B, Arany E, Zaina S, Conkell S, Graham CF. Increased and persistent circulating insulin-like growth factor II in neonatal transgenic mice suppresses developmental apoptosis in the pancreatic islets. *Endocrinology* 2000; **141**: 1151–7

8   Reddy S, Elliott RB. Ontogenic development of peptide hormones in the mammalian fetal pancreas. *Experientia* 1988; **44**: 1–9

9   Mally MI, Otonkosk T, Lopez AD, Haycock A. Developmental gene expression in the human fetal pancreas. *Pediatr Res* 1994; **36**: 537–44

10 Fowden AL. Pancreatic endocrine function and carbohydrate metabolism in the fetus. In: Abrecht E, Pepe GJ. (eds) *Research in Perinatal Medicine IV*. Ithaca, NY: Perinatology Press, 1985; 71–90

11 Fowden AL. Endocrine regulation of fetal growth. *Reprod Fertil Dev* 1995; **7**: 351–63

12 Lips JP, Acuk WJ, Crevels J, Eskes TK. Chronic hyperglycaemia and insulin concentrations in fetal lambs. *Am J Obstet Gynecol* 1988; **159**: 247–51

13 Dahri S, Reusen B, Remacle C, Hoet JJ. Nutritional influences on pancreatic development – potential links with non-insulin-dependent diabetes. *Proc Nutr Soc* 1995; **54**: 345–56

14 Aldoretta PW, Carver TD, Hay WW. Maturation of glucose stimulated insulin secretion in fetal sheep. *Biol Neonate* 1998; **73**: 375–86

15 Carver TD, Anderson SM, Aldoretta PW, Hay WW. Effect of low-level basal plus marked pulsatile hyperglycaemia on insulin secretion in fetal sheep. *Am J Physiol* 1996; **271**: E865–71

16 Godfrey KM, Robinson S, Hales CN, Barker DJP, Osmond C, Taylor KP. Nutrition in pregnancy and the concentrations of proinsulin, 32/33 split proinsulin, insulin and C-peptide in cord plasma. *Diabet Med* 1996; **13**: 868–73

17 Hales CN, Desai M, Ozanne SE, Crowther NJ. Fishing in the stream of diabetes: from measuring insulin to the control of fetal organogenesis. *Biochem Soc Trans* 1996; **24**: 341–50

18 Berney DM, Desai M, Palmer DJ *et al*. The effects of maternal protein deprivation on the fetal rat pancreas: major structural changes and their recuperation. *J Pathol* 1997; **183**: 109–15

19 Nielsen JH, Serup P. Molecular basis for islet development, growth and regeneration. *Curr Opin Endocrinol Diabetes* 1998; **5**: 97–107

20 Sander M, German S. The β cell transcription factors and development of the pancreas. *J Mol Med* 1997; **75**: 327–40

21 Offield MF, Jetton TL, Labosky PA *et al*. PDX-1 is required for pancreatic outgrowth and differentiation of the rostral duodenum. *Development* 1996; **122**: 983–95

22 Stoffers DA, Zinkin FT, Stanojevik V, Clarke WL, Habener JF. Pancreatic agenesis attributable to a single deletion in the human IPF-1 coding region. *Nat Genet* 1997; **15**: 106–10

23 Sosa-Pineda B, Chowdhury K, Torres M, Oliver G, Gruss P. The Pax-4 gene is essential for the differentiation of insulin-producing β-cells in mammalian pancreas. *Nature* 1997; **386**: 399–402

24 St-Onge L, Sosa-Pineda B, Chowdhury K, Mansouri A, Gruss P. Pax6 is required for differentiation of glucagon-producing cells in mouse pancreas. *Nature* 1997; **387**: 406–8

25 Velho G, Froguel P. Genetic, metabolic and clinical characteristics of maturity onset diabetes of the young. *Eur J Endocrinol* 1998; **138**: 233–9

26 Yamagata K, Furuta H, Oda N *et al*. Mutations in the hepatocyte nuclear factor 4 alpha gene in maturity-onset diabetes of the young (MODY1). *Nature* 1996; **384**: 468–70

27 Froguel P, Vaxillaire M, Sun F *et al*. Close linkage of glucokinase locus on chromosome 7p to early-onset non-insulin-dependent diabetes mellitus. *Nature* 1992; **356**: 162–4

28 Velho G, Blanché H, Vaxillaire M *et al*. Identification of 14 new glucokinase mutations and description of the clinical profile of 42 MODY-2 families. *Diabetologia* 1997; **40**: 217–24

29 Vaxillaire M, Rouard M, Yamagata K *et al*. Identification of nine novel mutations in the hepatocyte nuclear factor 1 alpha gene associated with maturity onset diabetes of the young

(MODY 3). *Hum Mol Genet* 1997; **6**: 583–6

30 Stoffers DA, Ferrer J, Clarke WL, Habener JF. Early-onset type 2 diabetes mellitus (MODY4) linked to IPF1. *Nat Genet* 1997; **17**: 138–9

31 Byrne MM, Sturis J, Menzel S *et al.* Altered insulin secretory responses to glucose in diabetic and nondiabetic subjects with mutations in the diabetes mellitus susceptibility gene MODY on chromosome 12. *Diabetes* 1996; **45**: 1503–10

32 Byrne MM, Sturis J, Fajans SS *et al.* Altered secretory responses to glucose in subjects with a mutation in the MODY1 gene on chromosome 20. *Diabetes* 1995; **44**: 699–704

33 Herman WH, Fajans SS, Ortiz FJ *et al.* Abnormal insulin secretion, not insulin resistance, is the genetic or primary defect of MODY in the RW pedigree. *Diabetes* 1994; **43**: 40–6

34 Carver TD, Anderson SM, Aldoretta PE, Esler AL, Hay WW. Glucose suppression of insulin secretion in chronically hyperinsulinaemic fetal sheep. *Pediatr Res* 1995; **38**: 754–62

35 Kervan A, Guillaume M, Frost A. The endocrine pancreas of the fetus from diabetic pregnant rats. *Diabetologia* 1975; **15**: 387–93

36 Terauchi Y, Kubota N, Tamemoto H *et al.* Insulin effect during embryogenesis determines fetal growth: A possible molecular link between birth weight and susceptibility to type 2 diabetes. *Diabetes* 2000; **49**: 82–6

37 Cherif H, Rensens B, Ahn MJ, Hoet JJ, Remacle C. Effect of taurine on the insulin secretion of islets of fetus from dams fed a low protein diet. *Endocrinology* 1998; **159**: 341-8

38 Dahri S, Snoeck A, Reuse-Billen B, Remacle C, Hoet JJ. Islet function in offspring of mothers on low protein diet during late gestation. *Diabetes* 1991; **40 (Suppl 2)**: 115–20

39 Ozanne SE, Hales CN. The long term consequences of intra-uterine protein malnutrition for glucose metabolism. *Proc Nutr Soc* 1999; **58**: 615–9

40 Petrik J, Reusens B, Avany E *et al.* A low protein diet alters the balance of islet cell replication and apoptosis in the fetus and is associated with a reduced pancreatic expression of insulin-like growth factor-II. *Endocrinology* 1999; **140**: 4861–73

41 Snoeck A, Remacle C, Reises B, Hoet JJ. Effect of a low protein diet during pregnancy on the fetal rat endocrine pancreas. *Biol Neonate* 1990; **57**: 107–18

42 Hoet JJ, Hanson MA. Intrauterine nutrition: its importance during critical periods for cardiovascular and endocrine development. *J Physiol* 1999; **514**: 617–27

43 Fowden AL, Forhead AJ. The role of hormones in intrauterine development. In: Barker DJP. (ed) *Fetal Origins of Cardiovascular and Like Disease*. New York: Marcel Decker, 2000; 199–228

44 Fowden AL, Li J, Forhead AJ. Glucocorticoids and the preparation for life after birth: are there long-term consequences of the life insurance? *Proc Nutr Soc* 1998; **57**: 113–22

45 Hill DJ, Petrik J, Arany E. Growth factors and the regulation of fetal growth. *Diabetes Care* 1998; **21 (Suppl 2)**: B60–9

46 Oberg-Welsh C, Welsh M. Effects of certain growth factors on in vitro maturation of rat fetal islet-like structures. *Pancreas* 1996; **12**: 334–9

47 Yi ES, Yin S, Harclerode DL *et al.* Keratinocyte growth factor induces pancreatic ductal epithelial proliferation. *Am J Pathol* 1994; **145**: 80–5

48 Nguyen HQ, Danilenko DM, Bucay N *et al.* Expression of keratinocyte growth factor in embryonic liver of transgenic mice causes changes in epithelial growth and differentiation resulting in polycystic kidneys and other organ malformations. *Oncogene* 1996; **12**: 2109–19

49 Arany E, Petrik J, Hill DJ. Fibroblast growth factors and beta cell neogenesis in the developing rat pancreata. *J Endocrinol* 1998; **156 (Suppl)**: P104

50 Rubin JS, Bottaro DP, Chedid M *et al.* Keratinocyte growth factor. *Cell Biol Int* 1995; **19**: 399–411

51 Hill DJ, Hogg J, Peptrik J, Arany EI, Hai VK. Cellular distribution and ontogeny of insulin-like growth factors (IGFs) and IGF binding protein messenger RNAs and peptides in developing rat pancreas. *J Endocrinol* 1999; **160**: 305–17

52 Hiettinen PJ, Otonkoski J, Voutilainer R. Insulin-like growth factor-II and transforming growth-factor alpha in developing human fetal pancreatic islets. *J Endocrinol* 1993; **138**: 127–36

53 Petrik J, Pell JM, Arany E *et al.* Over expression on insulin-like growth factor II in transgenic mice is associated with pancreatic islet cell hyperplasia. *Endocrinology* 1999; **140**: 2353–63

54 Iglesisa-Barreiva V, Ahn M-T, Reutens B, Dahri S, Hoet JJ, Remacle C. Pre and postnatal low protein diet affect pancreatic islet blood flow and insulin release in adult rats. *Endocrinology* 1996; **137**: 3797–801

55 Ozanne SE, Smith GD, Tikerpae J, Hales CN. Altered regulation of hepatic glucose output in male offspring of protein-malnourished rat dams. *Am J Physiol* 1996; **270**: E559–64

56 Hogg J, Han VR, Clemmons DR, Hill DJ. Interactions of nutrients, insulin-like growth factors (IGFs) and IGF-binding proteins in the regulation DNA synthesis by isolated fetal rat islets of Langerhans. *J Endocrinol* 1993; **138**: 401–12

57 Desai M, Byrne CD, Meeran K, Martinez ND, Bloom SR, Hales CN. Regulation of hepatic enzymes and insulin levels in offspring of rat dams fed a reduced protein diet. *Am J Physiol* 1997; **273**: G899–904

58 Nyirendi MJ, Lindsay RS, Kenyon CJ, Burchell A, Seckl JR. Glucocorticoid exposure in late gestation permanently programs rat hepatic phosphoenolpyruvate carboxykinase and glucocorticoid receptor expression and cause glucose intolerance in adult offspring. *J Clin Invest* 1998; **101**: 2174–81

59 Hunziker E, Stein M. Nestin-expressing cell in the pancreatic islets of Langerhans. *Biochem Biophys Res Commun* 2000; **271**: 116–9

60 German MS, Wang J. The insulin gene contains multiple transcriptional elements that respond to glucose. *Mol Cell Biol* 1994; **14**: 4067–75

61 Dunger DB, Ong KKL, Huxtable SJ et al. Association of the INS VNTR with size at birth. *Nat Genet* 1998; **19**: 98–100

62 Ong KKL, Phillips DIW, Fall C et al. The insulin gene VNTR, type 2 diabetes and birth weight. *Nat Genet* 1999; **21**: 262–3

63 Guilliam M-T, Hummler E, Schaerer E et al. Early diabetes and abnormal postnatal pancreatic islet development in mice lacking GLUT-2. *Nat Genet* 1997; **17**: 327–30

64 Hattersley AJ, Tooke J. The fetal insulin hypothesis in an alternate explanation of the association of low birthweight with diabetes and vascular disease. *Lancet* 1999; **353**: 1789–92

65 Garafano A, Czernillow P, Breant B. Effect of ageing on beta cell mass and function in rats malnourished during the perinatal period. *Diabetologia* 1999; **42**: 711–8

66 Jorns A, Tiedge M, Lenzen S. Nutrient-dependent distribution of insulin and glucokinase immunoactivities in rat pancreatic beta cells. *Virchows Arch* 1999; **434**: 75–82

67 Kornel L, Prancan AV, Kanamarlapudi N, Hynes J, Kuzianik E. Study on the mechanisms of glucocorticoid induced hypertension: glucocorticoid increase transmembrane Ca^{2+} influx in vascular smooth muscle *in vitro*. *Endocr Res* 1995; **21**: 203–10

68 Rorsman P, Arklanmar P, Bokvist K et al. Failure of glucose to elicit a normal secretary response in fetal pancreatic beta cells results from glucose insensitivity of the ATP regulated K^+ channels. *Proc Natl Acad Sci USA* 1989; **86**: 4505–9

69 Szep Y, Iqbal Z. Glucocorticoid action on depolarization dependent calcium influx in brain synaptosomes. *Neuroendocrinology* 1994; **59**: 457–65

Metabolic programming in animals

Susan E Ozanne

Department of Clinical Biochemistry, University of Cambridge, Cambridge, UK

A large number of epidemiological studies have revealed that there is a relationship between early growth restriction and the subsequent development of type 2 diabetes or the metabolic syndrome. The mechanistic basis of this relationship and the relative roles played by genes and the environment remains the subject of much current debate. Animal models of early growth restriction have been developed in an attempt to understand its relationship with adult disease and to provide insight into the underlying molecular mechanisms. These models show many features of the metabolic syndrome. In the maternal protein restriction model, insulin resistance and hypertension is observed. The uterine artery ligation model shows obesity in adulthood. This provides strong evidence that alterations in the fetal environment can lead to diabetes in adult life.

The term programming has been used to describe the process whereby a stimulus or insult when applied at a critical or sensitive period of development results in a long-term or permanent effect on the structure or function of the organism[1]. The long-term effects of an insult during a critical period of development has been recognised for many years. However, over the last decade, immense interest in programming has been prompted by the results of a large number of epidemiological studies which have shown that there is a relationship between early growth restriction and the subsequent development of adult degenerative diseases such as type 2 diabetes, ischaemic heart disease and hypertension[2]. Little is known about the mechanistic basis of this relationship or the relative role of genetic and environmental factors. Extensive genomic scans have been unsuccessful in identifying universal diabetes susceptibility genes/polymorphisms. However, recent studies have identified rare mutations in the glucokinase gene which are associated with a reduced birth weight and the development of maturity-onset diabetes of the young (*see* Frayling & Hattersley, this issue)[3]. The importance of environmental factors has been demonstrated by a number of human studies. A study of twins in Denmark revealed that, in monozygotic twin pairs who were discordant for diabetes, the diabetic twin had a significantly lower birth weight than the normoglycaemic twin[4]. In addition, studies of individuals exposed *in utero* to famine during the Dutch hunger winter have revealed that poor maternal

Correspondence to:
Dr S E Ozanne,
Department of Clinical
Biochemistry (Level 4),
Addenbrooke's Hospital,
Hills Road, Cambridge
CB2 2QR, UK

nutrition, especially during the last trimester of pregnancy, leads to growth restriction of the fetus and is associated with poor glucose tolerance and insulin resistance[5].

In an attempt to understand the molecular basis of the relationship between early growth restriction and development of subsequent disease, animal models have been developed. There are a number of insults during pregnancy that have been shown to result in growth restriction in various species. These include both nutritional and hormonal insults as well as surgical interventions.

Nutritional models of early growth restriction

Maternal low protein

The maternal low protein model is one of the most extensively studied models of early growth restriction[6]. There are a striking number of parallels between findings from this model and those from studies of individuals with type 2 diabetes and/or the metabolic syndrome (Table 1). This low protein rat model has been used for a number of years and involves feeding rats a low (5–8%) protein diet during pregnancy which results in growth restriction of the offspring[7]. If such offspring are cross-fostered to mothers being fed a control (20%) protein diet during lactation, they rapidly gain weight such that by weaning (21 days of age) these recuperated offspring have similar body weights to controls. This catch-up growth appears to have a detrimental effect on longevity, resulting in premature death which is associated with accelerated loss of kidney telomeric DNA[8]. The detrimental effect of catch-up growth has also been reported in human populations. In Sweden, it has been shown that men who were born small but who grew to above average height have raised blood pressure[9]. More recently it has been shown that catch up growth in a Finnish cohort is associated with increased death from cardiovascular disease[10].

Table 1 Similarities between the low protein rat model and human metabolic syndrome

Physical features	Low birth weight
	Short stature
Whole body characteristics	Diabetes
	Insulin resistance
	Hypertension
Tissue characteristics	Altered regulation of hepatic glucose output
	Depot-selective adipocyte insulin resistance

Permanent growth restriction results if maternal protein restriction is continued during lactation even when the offspring themselves are weaned onto a control diet[7]. In young adult life, these offspring have a significantly better glucose tolerance than controls[11]. However, early growth restricted offspring undergo a greater age-dependent loss of glucose tolerance such that by 15 months of age glucose tolerance is significantly worse than that of controls[12]. This is associated with insulin resistance. In addition to an age-dependent loss of glucose tolerance, maternal protein restriction has been shown to be associated with hypertension[13]. It has been suggested that this hypertension may be related to changes in both kidney structure and the activity of the renin-angiotensin system[13]. Obesity and maternal protein restriction when combined have an independent and additive effect on blood pressure[14].

The long-term effects of maternal protein restriction on the structure and function of individual organs have also been investigated. Most of the early studies focused on the effect of early protein restriction on the development of the endocrine pancreas (see Bertram & Hanson, this issue). β-Cell proliferation and islet size was shown to be significantly reduced in the head of the pancreas of neonates from dams fed a low protein diet during pregnancy[15]. Apoptosis of β-cells was also shown to be increased in 14-day-old low protein neonates[16] and islet vascularization[15] was significantly reduced in the head and tail of the pancreas of these offspring. The studies were extended to determine if these structural changes were associated with any changes in insulin secretion. No differences in basal secretion were observed. However, islets from 21.5-day-old fetuses of low protein mothers had a reduced secretory response to both leucine and arginine *in vitro*[17]. Subsequently, it was shown that a defect in glucose-stimulated insulin secretion from islets of adult low protein offspring is only observed when an additional dietary insult such as high fat or sucrose feeding is introduced postnatally[18]. This supports the hypothesis that it is an imbalance between the environment in early and adult life that may lead to diseases such as type 2 diabetes and thus make nutritional intervention programmes a realistic possibility. Indeed, recent studies have demonstrated that supplementing the mothers' diet with taurine prevents the impaired insulin secretion normally observed in fetuses of low protein-fed dams[19]. The precise time window available for such an effect of taurine requires further investigation.

Maternal protein restriction has also been shown to have long-term effects on insulin sensitive tissues. In the liver, this includes both structural and functional changes. It has been observed that low protein offspring have larger hepatic lobules compared to controls[20]. *Ex vivo* liver perfusions of 3-month-old male animals have shown that low protein offspring are relatively resistant to the ability of glucagon to stimulate hepatic glucose output compared to controls[21]. This glucagon resistance is related to a reduction in expression of glucagon receptors[21]. These studies also revealed that livers of low protein offspring exhibited an anomalous response to insulin, with the hormone initially stimulating hepatic glucose output[21]. A similar paradoxical response to insulin has been reported in subjects with type 2 diabetes[22] and in young Aborigines[23] (a population where a large number of individuals develop diabetes).

In young adult life, skeletal muscle from low protein offspring is more sensitive to insulin in terms of its ability to stimulate glucose uptake[24]. This increased sensitivity is related to increased expression of insulin receptors and presumably, at least in part, contributes to their better glucose tolerance at this age compared to controls.

Detailed analysis of adipocytes from low protein and control offspring have identified potential markers of early growth restriction[25]. Adipocytes isolated from young adult, low protein offspring have an elevated basal and insulin-stimulated glucose uptake and increased levels of insulin receptor[25]. Over the last decade, our understanding of the way in which insulin signals to metabolic actions has increased enormously[26]. Following insulin binding, the insulin receptor becomes autophosphorylated on tyrosine residues and subsequently phosphorylates a number of insulin receptor substrates including insulin receptor substrate (IRS)-1. A number of downstream signalling elements are able to bind to phosphorylated insulin receptor substrates and become activated. One such enzyme is phosphatidylinositide (PI)-3-kinase which has been shown by inhibitor studies to be necessary for both the action of insulin to stimulate glucose uptake and to inhibit lipolysis[27]. Consistent with the observed changes in glucose uptake, adipocytes from 3-month-old low protein offspring have an elevated basal and insulin-stimulated IRS-1 associated PI-3-kinase activity. However, despite having elevated levels of PI-3-kinase activity, these adipocytes are resistant to the antilipolytic action of insulin[28]. This observation was at first surprising, but a more detailed analysis of PI-3-kinase has suggested a potential mechanistic basis of these findings. PI-3-kinase is a heterodimeric enzyme which consists of a regulatory subunit (p85) and a catalytic subunit (p110)[27]. Two isoforms (p110α and p110β) of the catalytic subunit are present in adipocytes[27]. Early protein restriction leads to a dramatic reduction in expression of p110β while expression of p110α remains unchanged[25]. Little is known about the functional differences between these two isoforms. However, the existence of differentially regulated isoforms with divergent signalling roles would allow the cell to adjust its metabolic status in response to its environment. Measurement of the relative expression levels of these two isoforms of p110 could provide important information on the success of a fetus at achieving its growth potential. However, data on the expression of these proteins in human growth restriction are not currently available. This information may prove to be difficult to obtain, as studies in the low protein offspring[28] and in humans[29] with metabolic syndrome have both suggested that resistance to the antilipolytic action of insulin is depot specific with intra-abdominal fat being resistant and subcutaneous fat (the most available depot for biopsy) remaining relatively insulin sensitive.

Maternal calorie restriction

The effects of various regimens of total food restriction have been studied by a number of investigators. Early studies focused on the long-term effects of short-term food restriction in early postnatal life[30]. It was shown that feeding rats a calorie restricted diet between 3–6 weeks of age caused an impairment of insulin secretory response that was still evident at 12 weeks of age[30]. More recently, the focus of studies has been on the long-term effects of maternal calorie restriction. Severe food restriction (to only 30% of *ad libitum* intake) during pregnancy has been shown to induce severe growth restriction in the fetus[31]. In adulthood, these offspring have slightly elevated systolic blood pressures[31] and increased fasting plasma insulin concentrations[32] compared to control offspring. These offspring have also been shown to have increased food intakes compared to control offspring. This hyperphagia was shown to increase with age and could be amplified by hypercaloric nutrition. This finding is consistent with findings in humans which suggest that early growth restriction is associated with adult central obesity[33]. Less severe food restriction (to 50% of *ad libitum* intake) from day 15 of pregnancy to weaning has been shown to result in insulinopaenia and an age-dependent loss of glucose tolerance which is apparent in 12-month-old male offspring[34].

Maternal iron restriction

Iron deficiency is a common nutritional problem in humans and is especially prevalent in pregnant women. It has been shown that feeding rats an iron-deficient diet during pregnancy leads to anaemia and growth restriction of the fetus[35]. The long-term effects of such maternal iron-deficient anaemia are not well documented. A number of studies have shown that the offspring have decreased iron concentrations in brain tissue which can not be normalised by iron treatment after weaning[36]. In addition, behavioural differences have been noted in these offspring[36]. In early postnatal life (day 20), heart weights of the offspring of anaemic dams have been shown to be increased suggesting an alteration in their cardiovascular development[37]. This, however, is paradoxically associated with decreased systolic blood pressure compared to control pups at this age[37]. Chronic fetal anaemia in the sheep has been shown to be associated with similar cardiac hypertrophy and a lowering of mean arterial pressure in ovine fetuses around day 133 of gestation[38]. This is suggested to be related to a decrease in total peripheral resistance. In the rat model, changes in blood pressure have been reported to be age-dependent. Despite having lower systolic blood pressure on day 20 of postnatal life, by day 40 the pressures of offspring of iron-deficient dams were reported to be significantly elevated compared to controls[37]. The mechanistic basis of this elevation of blood pressure is not known.

Hormonal insults

Glucocorticoid exposure

It has been known for over 20 years that glucocorticoid treatment during pregnancy in both humans and animals causes a reduction in birth weight[39]. However, it is only in the last decade, in light of the epidemiological data linking low birth weight to adult disease, that the long-term consequences of prenatal glucocorticoid exposure have been investigated[40]. Offspring that have been exposed to excess prenatal glucocorticoids undergo catch-up growth postnatally and it has been shown that body weights have normalised by weaning (3 weeks of age) in the rat. Findings in such adult offspring are consistent with the hypothesis that rapid postnatal catch-up growth is deleterious to adult health. Fetal glucocorticoid overexposure in rats has been shown to be associated with elevated blood pressure[41] and raised blood glucose levels[42] in adulthood. This phenotypic outcome is similar to that of the low protein model and it has been suggested that fetal glucocorticoid overexposure may be a common mechanism linking maternal environmental factors with fetal growth and programming[40]. This suggestion in based on the observation that dietary protein restriction during rat pregnancy reduces 11β-hydroxysteroid dehydrogenase 2 activity[40]. This enzyme forms a placental 'barrier' which catalyses the rapid metabolism of active physiological glucocorticoids to inert 11-keto forms, thus minimising fetal exposure to glucocorticoids[40].

Surgical intervention

Uterine artery ligation

Impaired utero–placental perfusion with an associated reduction in placental transport of nutrients is thought to be responsible for a large number of cases of intra-uterine growth restriction in humans[43]. Reduction in placental blood flow and transport and a consequent restriction of fetal growth can be produced in the rat by uterine artery ligation in late gestation[44]. Most studies on this model to date have focused on the offspring during fetal and early postnatal life. It has been shown that at birth and at 2 weeks of age, growth-retarded offspring have reduced nephron number[45]. This nephron deficit was associated with impaired renal function at 2 weeks of age despite an apparent large compensatory hypertrophy of nephrons in these animals[45]. A more molecular analysis of skeletal muscle from fetuses and 21-day-old offspring following uterine artery ligation has revealed that this mode of growth restriction is associated with changes in both mitochondrial gene expression and function. In fetal life, mRNA levels of the mitochondrial proteins NADH-ubiquinone-oxidoreductase subunit 4L, subunit C of the F_1F_0 ATP synthase and adenine nucleotide translocator 1 were all reduced[46]. In contrast, by day 21 postnatally, mRNA levels of all three proteins were reduced compared to controls[46]. This was associated with a reduced skeletal muscle mitochondrial $NAD^+/NADH$ ratio, indicative of an alteration in mitochondrial function[46].

One study of adult offspring (3–4 months of age) has suggested that this method of early growth restriction is not associated with hypertension[47]. This contrasts with the data obtained from offspring which were growth restricted by maternal protein restriction, maternal calorie restriction, maternal iron restriction or maternal dexamethasone treatment. This suggests that intra-uterine growth restriction *per se* is not sufficient to cause elevated blood pressure in adulthood. Subtle differences such as the timing of the insult during pregnancy and the composition of the adult diet may also be important. In terms of glucose tolerance, effects of such placental insufficiency appear to be sex specific[47]. Young adult male offspring were shown to have similar fasting blood glucose and plasma insulin levels compared to controls. In addition, glucose tolerance was not related to birth weight[47]. In contrast, in female offspring, growth restriction was associated with increased fasting blood glucose levels. Fasting plasma insulin levels were unaltered by growth restriction suggesting a degree of insulin resistance in growth restricted animals[47]. Early growth restriction in females was also associated with impaired glucose tolerance and lower insulin secretion during a glucose tolerance test. This suggests that, in female rats, intra-uterine growth restriction caused by uterine artery ligation is associated with an impaired regulation of insulin secretion by glucose.

Future prospects

One of the major problems in applying the data obtained from the epidemiological studies to clinical practice is in identifying individuals who have been growth restricted *in utero*. Birth weight is only a crude index of early growth (*see* Barker, this issue) and reveals nothing about the success of a fetus at achieving its growth potential. In addition, animal and human studies have shown that certain insults during pregnancy can have long-term effects on the metabolism of the offspring in the absence of an effect on birth weight. A key area of future research will thus be to identify markers of early growth restriction which may be of future diagnostic use as early predictors of adult disease. It is not clear if these markers will be specific to individual causes of growth restriction or if these markers will be shared between numerous forms of growth restriction.

References

1   Lucas A. Programming by early nutrition in man. In: Bock GR, Whelan J. (eds) *The Childhood Environment and Adult Disease* (CIBA Foundation Symposium 156). Chichester: Wiley, 1991; 38–55

2   Philips DIW, Hales CN. The intrauterine environment and susceptibility to non-insulin dependent diabetes and the insulin resistance syndrome. In: Marshall SM, Home PD, Rizza RA. (eds) *The Diabetes Annual*, vol 10. Amsterdam: Elsevier, 1996; 1–13

3   Hattersley AT, Beards F, Ballantyne E, Appleton M, Harvey R, Ellard S. Mutations in the glucokinase gene of the fetus result in reduced birthweight. *Nat Genet* 1998; **19**: 268–70

4   Poulsen P, Vaag AA, Kyvik KO, Moller-Jensen D, Beck-Nielson H. Low birthweight is associated with NIDDM in discordant monozygotic and dizygotic twin pairs. *Diabetologia* 1997; **40**: 439–46

5   Ravelli ACJ, van der Meulen JHP, Michels RPJ *et al.* Glucose tolerance in adults after prenatal exposure to famine. *Lancet* 1998; **351**: 173–7

6   Ozanne SE, Hales CN. The long term consequences of intra-uterine protein malnutrition on glucose metabolism. *Proc Nutr Soc* 1999; **58**: 615–9

7   Desai M, Crowther NJ, Lucas A, Hales CN. Organ-selective growth in the offspring of protein restricted mothers. *Br J Nutr* 1996; **76**: 591–603

8   Jennings BJ, Ozanne SE, Dorling MW, Hales CN. Early growth determines longevity in male rats and may be related to telomere shortening in the kidney. *FEBS Lett* 1999; **448**: 4–9

9   Leon D, Koupilova I, Lithell HO *et al.* Failure to realise growth potential *in utero* and adult obesity in relation to blood pressure in 50 year old Swedish men. *BMJ* 1996; **312**: 401–6

10 Eriksson JG, Forsen T, Tuomilehto J, Winter PD, Osmond C, Barker DJP. Catch-up growth in childhood and death from coronary heart disease: longitudinal study. *BMJ* 1999; **13**: 427–31

11 Shepherd PR, Crowther NJ, Desai M, Hales CN, Ozanne SE. Altered adipocyte properties in the offspring of protein malnourished rats. *Br J Nutr* 1997; **78**: 121–9

12 Hales CN, Desai M, Ozanne SE, Crowther NJ. Fishing in the stream of diabetes: from measuring insulin to the control of fetal organogenesis. *Biochem Soc Trans* 1996; **24**: 341–50

13 Langley Evans SC, Sherman RC, Welham SJ, Nwagwu MO, Gardner DS, Jackson AA. Intrauterine programming of hypertension: the role of the renin-angiotensin system. *Biochem Soc Trans* 1999; **27**: 88–93

14 Petry CJ, Ozanne SE, Wang CL, Hales CN. Early protein restriction and obesity independently induce hypertension in year old rats. *Clin Sci* 1997; **93**: 147–52

15 Snoeck A, Remacle C, Reusens B, Hoet JJ. Effect of a low protein diet during pregnancy on the fetal rat endocrine pancreas. *Biol Neonate* 1990; **57**: 107–18

16 Petrik J, Reusens B, Arany E *et al.* A low protein diet alters the balance of islet cell replication and apoptosis in the fetal and neonatal rat and is associated with a reduced pancreatic expression of insulin-like growth factor-II. *Endocrinology* 1999; **140**: 4861–73

17 Dahri S, Snoeck A, Reusens-Billen B, Remacle C, Hoet JJ. Islet function in offspring of mothers on low-protein diet during gestation. *Diabetes* 1991; **40**: 115–20

18 Wilson MR, Hughes SJ. The effect of maternal protein deficiency during pregnancy and lactation on glucose tolerance and pancreatic islet function in adult rat offspring. *J Endocrinol* 1997; **27**: 177–85

19 Cherif H, Reusens B, Ahn MT, Hoet JJ, Remacle C. Effects of taurine on the insulin secretion of rat fetal islets from dams fed a low-protein diet. *J Endocrinol* 1998; **159**: 341–8

20 Burns SP, Desai M, Cohen RD *et al*. Gluconeogenesis, glucose handling and structural changes in livers of the adult offspring of rats partially deprived of protein during pregnancy and lactation *J Clin Invest* 1997; **100**: 1768–74

21 Ozanne SE, Smith GD, Tikerpae J, Hales CN. Altered regulation of hepatic glucose output in the male offspring of protein malnourished rat dams. *Am J Physiol* 1996; **270**: E55–64

22 Frank JW, Saslow SB, Camilleri M, Thomforde GM, Dinneen S, Rizza RA. Mechanism of accelerated gastric emptying of liquids and hyperglycaemia in patients with type II diabetes mellitus. *Gastroenterology* 1995; **109**: 755–65

23 Proietto J, Nankervis AJ, Traianedes K, Rosella G, O'Dea K. Identification of early metabolic defects in diabetes-prone Australian Aborigines. *Diabetes Res Clin Pract* 1992; **17**: 217–26

24 Ozanne SE, Wang CL, Coleman N, Smith GD. Altered muscle insulin sensitivity in the male offspring of protein malnourished rats. *Am J Physiol* 1996; **271**: E1128–34

25 Ozanne SE, Nave BT, Wang CL, Shepherd PR, Prins J, Smith GD. Poor fetal nutrition causes long term changes in expression of insulin signalling components in adipocytes. *Am J Physiol* 1997; **273**: E46–51

26 Virkamaki A, Ueki K, Kahn CR. Protein-protein interaction in insulin signaling and the molecular mechanisms of insulin resistance. *J Clin Invest* 1999; **103**: 931–43

27 Shepherd PR, Withers DJ, Siddle K. Phosphoinositide 3-kinase: the key switch mechanism in insulin signalling. *Biochem J* 1998; **333**: 471–90

28 Ozanne SE, Wang CL, Dorling MW, Petry CJ. Dissection of the metabolic actions of insulin in adipocytes from early growth retarded male rats. *J Endocrinol* 1999; **162**: 313–9

29 Arner P. Adipose tissue – the link between obesity and insulin resistance [Abstract]. *Proceedings of the British Hyperlipidaemic Association Scientific Workshop on Insulin Resistance*. London: Royal College of Surgeons, 1999

30 Swenne I, Grace CJ, Milner RDG. Persistent impairment of insulin secretory response to glucose in adult rats after limited period of protein calorie malnutrition early in life. *Diabetes* 1987; **36**: 454–8

31 Woodall SM, Johnston BM, Breier BH, Gluckman PD. Chronic maternal under-nutrition in the rat leads to delayed postnatal growth and elevated blood pressure of offspring. *Pediatr Res* 1996; **40**: 438–43

32 Vickers MH, Breier MH, Cutfield WS, Hofman PL, Gluckman PD. Fetal origins of hyperphagia, obesity and hypertension and postnatal amplification by hypercaloric nutrition. *Am J Physiol* 2000; **279**: E83–7

33 Law CM, Barker DJ, Osmond C, Fall CH, Simmonds SJ. Early growth and abdominal fatness in adult life. *J Epidemiol Community Health* 1992; **46**: 184–6

34 Garofano A, Czernichow P, Breant B. Effect of ageing on beta cell mass and function in rats malnourished during the perinatal period. *Diabetologia* 1999; **42**: 711–8

35 Shepard TH, Mackler B, Finch CA. Reproductive studies in the iron-deficient rat. *Teratology* 1980; **22**: 329–34

36 Felt BT, Lozoff B. Brain iron and behavior of rats are not normalized by treatment of iron deficiency anemia during early development. *J Nutr* 1996; **126**: 693–701

37 Crowe C, Dandekar P, Fox M, Dhingra K, Bennet L, Hanson MA. The effects of anaemia on heart, placenta and body weight, and blood pressure in fetal and neonatal rats. *J Physiol* 1995; **488**: 515–9

38 Martin CM, Yu AY, Jiang BH *et al*. Cardiac hypertrophy in chronically anemic fetal sheep: increased vascularization is associated with increased myocardial expression of vascular endothelial growth factor and hypoxia-inducible factor 1. *Am J Obstet Gynecol* 1998; **178**: 527–34

39 Reinisch JM, Simon NG, Karwo WG *et al*. Prenatal exposure to prednisone in humans and

animals retards intrauterine growth. *Science* 1978; **202**: 436–8

40 Seckl JR. Glucocorticoids, 11β-hydroxysteroid dehydrogenase and fetal programming. In: O'Brien PMS, Wheeler T, Barker DJP. (eds): *Fetal Programming. Influences on Development and Disease in Later Life*. London: Royal College of Obstetricians and Gynaecologists, 1999; 430–9

41 Benediktsson R, Lindsay RS, Noble J, Seckl JR, Edwards CRW. Glucocorticoid exposure *in utero*; a new model for adult hypertension. *Lancet* 1993; **341**: 339–41

42 Lindsay RS, Lindsay RM, Waddell BJ, Seckl JR. Prenatal glucocorticoid exposure leads to offspring hyperglycaemia in the rat; studies with the 11β-hydroxysteroid dehydrogenase inhibitor carbenoxolone. *Diabetologia* 1996; **39**: 1299–305

43 Bernstein I, Gabbe SG. Intrauterine growth restriction. In: Gabbe S, Niebyl J, Simpson J. (eds): *Obstetrics, Normal and Problem Pregnancies*. New York: Churchill Livingstone, 1996; 863–86

44 Wigglesworth JS. Fetal growth retardation. Animal model: uterine vessel ligation in the pregnant rat. *Am J Pathol* 1974; **77**: 347–50

45 Merlet-Benichou C, Gilbert T, Muffat-Joly M, Lelievre-Pegorier M, Leroy B. Intrauterine growth retardation leads to a permanent nephron deficit in the rat. *Pediatr Nephrol* 1994; **8**: 175–80

46 Lane RH, Chandorkar AK, Flozak AS, Simmons RA. Intrauterine growth retardation alters mitochondrial gene expression and function in fetal and juvenile rat skeletal muscle. *Pediatr Res* 1998; **43**: 563–70

47 Jansson T, Lambert GW. Effect of intrauterine growth restriction on blood pressure, glucose tolerance and sympathetic nervous system activity in the rat at 3–4 months of age. *J Hypertens* 1999; **17**: 1239–48

Programming other hormones that affect insulin

Christopher D Byrne

Endocrinology and Metabolism Unit, School of Medicine, University of Southampton, Southampton, UK

The metabolic syndrome is associated with a marked increase in risk of type 2 diabetes and atherosclerotic vascular disease (AVD). The mechanism responsible for the metabolic syndrome is uncertain, but recent evidence suggests that a combination of low birth weight and adult obesity is associated with a markedly increased prevalence. Insulin resistance is the cardinal feature of the metabolic syndrome. Several hormones, have modes of action that either potentiate or reduce the biological actions of insulin and, therefore, attenuate or induce insulin resistance. Since insulin action may be modified, these hormones potentially contribute to the pathogenesis of the metabolic syndrome.

The purpose of this review is to discuss programming of hormones that modulate insulin action. The review focuses on two major endocrine pathways: (i) glucocorticoid hormone action; and (ii) the growth hormone (GH)-insulin-like growth factor (IGF-1) axis, and discusses mechanisms linking abnormal activity of these pathways with reduced early growth, adult obesity and the metabolic syndrome

*Correspondence to:
Prof. Christopher D Byrne,
Endocrinology and
Metabolism Unit, South
Academic Block, Level D
(MP 811), Southampton
General Hospital,
Southampton
SO16 6YD, UK*

The metabolic syndrome (insulin resistance, hypertension, dyslipidaemia and glucose intolerance) is associated with a marked increase in risk of type 2 diabetes and atherosclerotic vascular disease (AVD). The central feature of this syndrome is insulin resistance. The pathogenesis of insulin resistance in subjects with the syndrome may explain much of the aetiology of type 2 diabetes and AVD in the industrialised world. The mechanism responsible for the metabolic syndrome is uncertain, but recent evidence suggests that a combination of low birth weight and adult obesity is associated with a markedly increased prevalence. Since features of the metabolic syndrome strongly predict AVD and type 2 diabetes[1,2], a mechanism is suggested linking reduced birth weight to type 2 diabetes and AVD. Development of the metabolic syndrome may be the mechanism linking reduced birth weight and adult obesity to type 2 diabetes and AVD. Prevalence of the metabolic syndrome is considerable in the industrialised world. Since features of the metabolic syndrome strongly predict type 2 diabetes and AVD, the population attributable risk for AVD and type 2 diabetes due to the metabolic syndrome is considerable.

Insulin resistance, or resistance to the normal physiological actions of insulin, is the cardinal feature of the metabolic syndrome. The explanation for a reduced biological action of insulin, despite markedly increased plasma insulin concentrations, remains uncertain. Factors countering the actions of insulin induce 'insulin resistance'. Several insulin antagonist hormones, such as glucocorticoid hormones, have modes of action that reduce the biological actions of insulin and, therefore, induce insulin resistance. Since insulin antagonist hormones induce insulin resistance, these hormones may contribute to the pathogenesis of the metabolic syndrome.

The purpose of this review is to discuss programming of hormones that modulate insulin action. The review will focus on two major endocrine pathways that have considerable impact on insulin sensitivity. There are three aims. First, to describe associations between reduced early growth and features of the metabolic syndrome in adulthood. Second, to illustrate mechanisms by which abnormal regulation of: (i) glucocorticoid hormone action; and (ii) the growth hormone (GH)-insulin-like growth factor (IGF-1) axis contribute to features of the metabolic syndrome. Finally, the third aim is to discuss associations between: (i) reduced early growth and glucocorticoid hormone action; and (ii) reduced early growth and the growth hormone (GH)-insulin-like growth factor (IGF-1) axis.

Low birth weight, adult obesity and prevalence of the metabolic syndrome

Low birth weight or other indices of sub-optimal fetal growth including stunting or thinness at birth are associated with an increased prevalence of atherosclerotic vascular disease (AVD) in adult life[3]. Low birth weight is associated with an increased prevalence of risk factors for AVD including type 2 diabetes, raised blood pressure and dyslipidaemia[4,5]. Glucose intolerance, raised blood pressure and dyslipidaemia tend to occur together as the metabolic syndrome[2] suggesting these features share a common pathogenesis. The potential shared aetiology has been referred to as the 'common soil' hypothesis[1]. Insulin resistance may underlie the 'common soil'. Low birth weight is associated with insulin resistance and the metabolic syndrome[5]; therefore, factors linked to low birth weight may be important in the pathogenesis of type 2 diabetes and AVD.

It has been shown that the prevalence of the metabolic syndrome was 6 times higher in men aged 65 years who weighed 5.5 1b (2.5 kg) or less at birth than in those who weighed 9.5 1b (4.3 kg) or more[5]. The relation

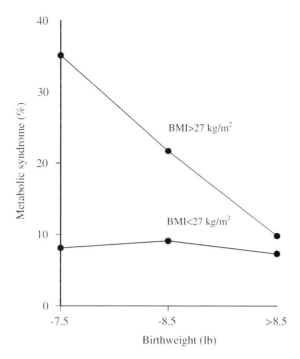

Fig. 1 Prevalence of features of the metabolic syndrome according to birth weight and adult body mass index (data from the Hertfordshire Study).

between birth size and the metabolic syndrome has now been observed in populations in Europe, North America and India[5-9]. These studies also show that adult obesity adds to the effect of reduced fetal growth in predicting the metabolic syndrome (Fig. 1).

More recent data suggest the presence of an interaction between reduced fetal growth and adult obesity such that the adverse effect of obesity is most marked in people who were also of low birth weight[10]. This is illustrated by data from the Hertfordshire study showing that adult obesity amplifies the strength of the association between low birth weight and features of the metabolic syndrome. Both the effects of low birth weight ($P < 0.001$), obesity ($P < 0.0001$), and the interaction between the two ($P = 0.01$) predicted the metabolic syndrome (defined as the presence of glucose intolerance or diabetes together with raised blood pressure and hyper-triglyceridaemia).

The hypothalamic–pituitary–adrenal axis

The metabolic syndrome and glucocorticoid hormone action

The mechanism by which glucocorticoid hormone action contributes to the metabolic syndrome is not fully elucidated, but many of the properties of glucocorticoid hormones are antagonistic to the actions of insulin, with important consequences for carbohydrate and lipid metabolism (for detailed review see Orth & Kovacs[11]). Glucocorticoid hormones also have a permissive effect to enhance actions of other insulin counter-regulatory hormones such as adrenaline and glucagon. For example, glucocorticoid hormones enhance the sensitivity of adipocytes to adrenaline to increase lipolysis, and skeletal muscle to release lactate. Glucocorticoid hormone acutely activates lipolysis in adipose tissue. Lipolytic activity and consequently plasma free fatty acid levels are reduced in adrenalectomised animals and return to normal within 2 h after glucocorticoid administration. This permissive effect may be mediated by altered sensitivity to other lipolytic hormones such as cate-cholamines and growth hormone, but the molecular mechanisms responsible are uncertain. Glucocorticoid hormones also exert chronic effects on lipid metabolism and one of the most striking observations in humans is the redistribution of body fat observed with chronic gluco-corticoid hormone excess. There is relative sparing of the extremities whereas there is marked accumulation of fat in a central distribution with increased fat also in the mesentery and omentum. It is possible that hyperinsulinaemia associated with insulin resistance contributes to this phenomenon, but the exact mechanism is still unclear.

Björntorp and others have suggested that a neuroendocrine disturbance involving the HPA axis may play an important part in the causation of the metabolic syndrome[12,13]. As patients with Cushing's syndrome develop a severe form of the metabolic syndrome with hypertension, insulin resistance, glucose intolerance, dyslipidaemia, and central obesity, it is an attractive idea that less profound disturbances of the HPA might underlie the metabolic syndrome. However, the published data supporting this idea are contradictory. Case-control and cross-sectional studies of people with-out pituitary or adrenal disease show that elevated plasma cortisol concentrations in morning samples are associated with high blood pressure, glucose intolerance, insulin resistance and hyperlipidaemia[14–16]. In contrast, other studies, particularly of centrally obese subjects, show a flattening of 24 h cortisol secretion with reduced morning cortisol concentrations[13,17–19]. Thus it is unlikely that altered activity of the HPA alone underlies the aetiology of the metabolic syndrome.

Recent evidence has suggested that altered cellular glucocorticoid hormone action may mediate features of the metabolic syndrome. Genetic polymorphisms of GR have been described that alter glucocorticoid hormone action and are associated with features of the metabolic syndrome[20]. However, recent studies suggest that the relative contribution of GR genotype to blood pressure is small[21]. This has lead to suggestions that tissue-specific molecular determinants of glucocorticoid hormone action may underlie the causative role of modest alterations in glucocorticoid hormone action in the pathogenesis of the metabolic syndrome[22,23].

We have recently obtained evidence that altered patterns of GR expression are associated with the metabolic syndrome. In a cross-sectional pilot study to investigate relationships between glucocorticoid hormone action and insulin sensitivity, we undertook hyperinsulinaemic euglycaemic clamps and skeletal muscle biopsies in 14 men. In muscle cell cultures established from these subjects, we have shown that GR mRNA levels are positively correlated with the degree of insulin resistance. GR mRNA levels were also positively correlated with BMI. These data indicate a strong link between tissue sensitivity to gluco-corticoid hormone and both resistance to insulin-mediated glucose uptake in skeletal muscle, and obesity. They suggest that increased tissue glucocorticoid sensitivity, mediated via increased GR expression, is likely to interact with factors that increase activity of the HPA axis. The net effect of increased HPA activity and tissue glucocorticoid sensitivity may contribute to the pathogenesis of the metabolic syndrome. In support of this idea, in another study systolic blood pressure was independently associated with both obesity (P <0.0001) and raised fasting plasma cortisol concentrations (P <0.001). Both factors interacted such that the relationship between fasting plasma cortisol concentrations and systolic blood pressure was strongest in the most obese subjects (P for interaction <0.05). A similar relationship was observed between synacthen respon-siveness, obesity and the metabolic syndrome. Risk of the metabolic syndrome was related to obesity (P <0.001) and synacthen responsiveness (P <0.001) and that the highest rates of the syndrome were observed in obese subjects who were most synacthen responsive.

Regulation of glucocorticoid hormone action

In physiological states, plasma glucocorticoid hormones circulate as plasma protein-hormone complexes with a corticosteroid-binding globulin. Free hormone diffuses into the cell and binds intracellular gluco-corticoid receptor (GR). Classically, GR is complexed to heat shock chaperone proteins (HSPs), such as HSP90. Two isoforms of GR have been identified, ligand binding GR-α and non-ligand binding GR-β. While GR-α mediates ligand-dependant hormone action, GR-β acts in a dominant negative manner to inhibit the actions of GR-α[24,25]. Moreover two functional classes of GR have also been identified, one with higher affinity for glucocorticoid hormone and another with lower affinity. After binding of hormone to cytosolic GR, there follows dissociation of heat shock proteins coupled with the formation of either homo- or heterodimers of GR isoforms and translocation of the complex to the nucleus. Ligand bound GR interacts with a number of transcript factors including AP1 and, through interactions between these GR-transcription factor complexes and complex glucocorticoid response elements, bring about regulation of gene expression. The nature of such regulation, *i.e.* whether up- or down-regulation of gene transcription also depends on the oncogenic components of AP1, *i.e.* the C-Jun/Fos ratio. Dynamic regulation of intracellular cortisol levels is mediated predominantly by the activity of the 11β-hydroxysteroid dehydrogenase (11β-HSD) enzymes, which can be regarded as pre-receptor signalling mechanisms regulating glucocorticoid hormone action through the interconversion of hormonally active cortisol and inactive cortisone. Clinical and experimental animal studies have revealed the expression of at least two kinetically distinct 11β-HSD isoforms which have been characterised[26,27]. Type 1 11β-HSD (11-HSD1) encodes relatively low affinity NADP/NADPH-dependent 11-dehydrogenase (cortisol to cortisone) and oxo-reductase (cortisone to cortisol) activity (K_m for cortisol = 1 μM; K_m for cortisone = 0.3 μM). In contrast, type 2 11β-HSD (11-HSD2) encodes high affinity NAD-dependent 11-dehydrogenase activity. The kinetic characteristics of these isoforms together with their distinct tissue-specific distribution suggests distinct physiological roles[28,29]. 11-HSD2 is localised predominantly to classical mineralocorticoid target tissues such as placenta and fetal tissues. 11-HSD2 confers aldosterone specificity on the mineralocorticoid receptor during postnatal life and tissue sensitivity to glucocorticoid during feto-placental development. In contrast, 11-HSD1 is localised to classical glucocorticoid target tissues. 11-HSD1 is thought to act predominantly as an 11-oxoreductase. 11-HSD1, therefore, regulates glucocorticoid hormone availability to GR.

Thus glucocorticoid hormone action results from an overall effect of many different factors. To summarise, these factors include: (i) activity of the HPA, (ii) regulators of pre-receptor glucocorticoid metabolism (*e.g.* 11HSD1 and 11HSD2); (iii) glucocorticoid hormone binding to GR; (iv) GR dimerisation; (v) translocation efficiency of the ligand-receptor complex to the nucleus; (vi) regulation of other transcription factors regulating GR; (vii) protein-DNA interactions with other transcription factors; and (viii) target gene response elements, modulating gene expression of gluco-corticoid-responsive genes.

Simplistically, these factors represent molecular determinants of gluco-corticoid hormone action. Each factor is theoretically able to modify gluco-corticoid function and, therefore, alter insulin sensitivity.

The early environment and glucocorticoid hormone action

Fetal overexposure to increased concentrations of glucocorticoids may influence development. Glucocorticoids slow fetal growth and may alter the size of the placenta, depending on the dose and timing of exposure[30]. These prenatal effects appear to persist after birth. For example, if a moderate dose of dexamethasone (a synthetic glucocorticoid that readily passes through the placenta) is given to a pregnant rat, it results in fetal growth retardation (average reduction ~14%), without affecting the gestation time or the viability of the fetus. A rise in systolic blood pressure in the adult offspring has been observed months after this exogenous glucocorticoid exposure[31]. Glucocorticoids have important effects on the maturation of tissues involved in blood pressure control. For example, development of catecholamine receptor expression is affected, and glucocorticoids influence second messenger systems in renal and vascular tissue. Glucocorticoids may also affect blood pressure by inducing growth factors, such as IGF or alternatively via indirect effects on carbohydrate and fat homeostasis[32]. In sheep, fetal blood pressure is increased when glucocorticoids are infused into the mother. The glucocorticoids affect the blood pressure directly by potentiating vasoconstrictor effects on the vasculature, and also by regulating the synthesis of catecholamines, nitric oxide and angiotensinogen, as well as having actions on the CNS[33].

Fetal cortisol levels are raised in intra-uterine growth retardation[34], and normally the fetus is protected from high maternal levels of physiological glucocorticoids (5–10-fold higher concentration than in the fetus) by the placental enzyme 11HSD2. 11HSD2 catalyses conversion of active cortisol to inactive cortisone. The efficiency of the placental barrier to maternal glucocorticoids varies considerably[35], and prenatal glucocorticoid exposure affects maturation of organs, an effect that may persist throughout life[34]. In rats, the lowest placental 11HSD2 activity, and therefore presumably the highest fetal exposure to maternal glucocorticoids, is associated with low birth weight fetuses, presumably as a result of cortisol retarding growth. It is these fetuses which develop the highest blood pressure, blood glucose and glucocorticoid levels in adulthood[31]. Treatment of pregnant rats with an 11HSD2 inhibitor, carbenoxolone, also reduces birth weight (by up to 20%) and raises blood pressure in the adult offspring (mean increase of 7–9 mmHg)[36]. However, the effect of fetal exposure to increased cortisol levels may differ depending upon the timing of exposure during gestation as intracellular glucocorticoid receptor is expressed in most fetal tissues from mid-gestation.

The mechanism controlling tissue glucocorticoid sensitivity is poorly understood. Dexamethasone administration in rat dams increases glucocorticoid sensitivity[37]. We have shown that nutritional manipulation is able to alter glucocorticoid sensitivity by modulating expression and function of glucocorticoid receptor (GR). Reduced maternal dietary protein intake during fetal and neonatal development produced a persistent reduction in hepatic GR expression and function in the adult offspring despite feeding these animals the normal diet from weaning until adulthood. We measured mRNA levels for three fibrinogen genes (using highly reproducible reverse transcriptase-PCR methodology developed in our laboratory)[38–40]. The three fibrinogen genes represent examples of glucocorticoid-responsive, but insulin-insensitive, target genes. Our results show that reducing maternal dietary protein intake during pregnancy and weaning not only resulted in reduced GR expression and function in the adult offspring, but also produced a parallel reduction in fibrinogen gene expression. These results suggest not only a decrease in tissue sensitivity to glucocorticoid hormone in the offspring, but also a parallel effect on expression of glucocorticoid responsive gene targets.

Animal experiments have shown that adverse influences in prenatal or early postnatal life permanently alter the biological and behavioural responses in the adult offspring by means of long-term changes in the set-point of central regulation of plasma glucocorticoid concentration. Exposure of pregnant rats to varieties of stress that include low protein diets, alcohol, physical restraint, or non-abortive maternal infections have shown that the offspring have increased HPA activity with increased stress-induced corticosteroid secretion in adult life[30,41–43]. It is thought that the effects of the stress may be mediated by excessive fetal exposure to glucocorticoid hormone resulting in persisting alterations in HPA activity. In support of this proposal, prenatal treatment of rats with dexamethasone, or the use of carbenoxolone to inhibit placental and fetal 11β-HSD to increase fetal glucocorticoid exposure, leads to permanently increased activity of the HPA in the offspring with increased circulating basal and stress-induced secretion of corticosterone[31,44]. This is probably effected in part by life-long alterations in the numbers of glucocorticoid receptors in the hippocampus, which is an important site of negative feedback of the HPA axis[45].

Recent evidence suggests that HPA programming may occur in association with reduced birth weight in humans. Among men aged 64 years, born in Hertfordshire, those who had lower birth weight had raised fasting plasma concentrations of cortisol. Timed fasting, plasma cortisol concentrations fell progressively from 408 nmol/1 among those whose birth weights were 5.5 1b (2.5 kg) or less to 309 nmol/1 among those who weighed 9.5 1b (4.3 kg) or more at birth, a trend independent of age and body mass index[36]. A study of a subset of 210 men from the original Hertfordshire cohort showed that low birth weight was associated with increased cortisol responsiveness to synthetic $ACTH_{1-24}$ (*P* trend for peak with birth weight = 0.03; *P* for trend of total response with birth weight = 0.009; Fig 2).

Similar relationships between birth size and fasting cortisol concentrations have also been demonstrated in two other populations, in Preston, UK, and in Adelaide, South Australia. The explanation for elevated plasma cortisol concentrations and response to ACTH in men with lower birth weight is unclear. Raised plasma cortisol concentrations

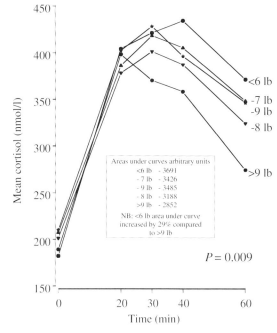

Fig. 2 Low dose synacthen test in 210 men showing cortisol responsiveness according to birthweight (data from the Hertfordshire Study).

may be due to: increased drive to ACTH secretion from higher centres, attenuated negative feedback, a change in adrenal sensitivity to ACTH, delayed peripheral metabolism of cortisol, or combinations of these factors.

To summarise, the available evidence suggests that a combination of factors causing (i) increased HPA activity with (ii) increased tissue sensitivity to glucocorticoid hormone, produce enhanced glucocorticoid hormone action and contribute to features of the metabolic syndrome. Increased glucocorticoid hormone action may be responsible, at least in part, for the association between low birth weight, adult obesity and the metabolic syndrome. A schematic representation is shown in Figure 3 illustrating regulation of the hypothalamic pituitary adrenal axis, glucocorticoid hormone action and development of the metabolic syndrome.

The growth hormone–insulin-like growth factor–IGF binding protein axis

Low growth rates *in utero* may alter the GH–IGF axis leading to reduced IGF-1 activity. This reduction in IGF-1 activity may cause altered insulin sensitivity in a tissue specific manner contributing to development of the metabolic syndrome.

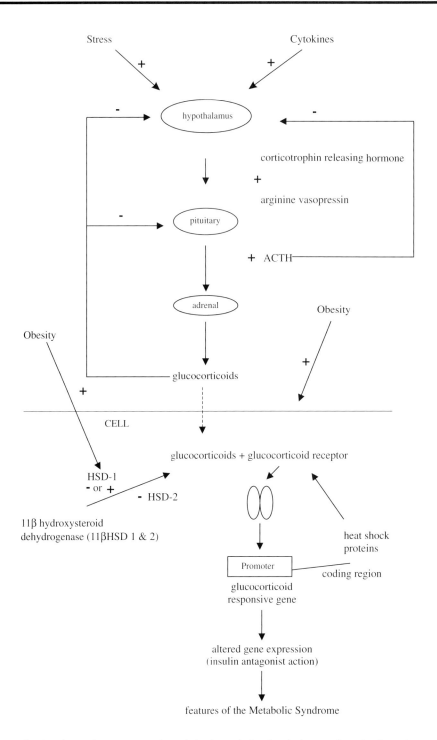

Fig. 3 Schematic representation of the hypothalamic–pituitary–adrenal axis and glucocorticoid hormone action.

The metabolic syndrome, the GH–IGF axis and insulin sensitivity

The metabolic syndrome is associated with changes throughout the GH–IGF axis, which may reduce IGF-1 activity. In obesity, GH secretion is diminished and clearance is enhanced, resulting in reduced free IGF-1 levels[46]. Serum IGF-1 is decreased in men with borderline hypertension and is associated with atherogenic lipid profiles in type 2 diabetes[47,48]. Serum IGFBP-1 is inversely correlated with a number of metabolic factors, including body mass index, lipid and insulin levels[48]. Increased BMI is associated with low overnight GH excretion[49]. Obesity is also associated with reduced nocturnal GH peaks and blunted GH responses to hypoglycaemia[50,51]. Detailed studies suggest that the low GH in obesity is a result of a combination of defects in GH secretion and clearance[50]. Since patients with adult GH deficiency develop insulin resistance, dyslipidaemia and central obesity, at the expense of lean tissue, less profound disturbances of the GH–IGF axis may underlie some of the features of the metabolic syndrome.

There are a number of possible mechanisms whereby alterations in the GH axis may influence cardiovascular risk in later life. In addition to its metabolic actions, GH has direct effects on myocardial growth and function and affects the expression of specific contractile proteins[52]. Both GH deficiency and GH excess are associated with abnormalities of cardiac function and recent evidence suggests that both low and high GH levels may be important predictors of cardiovascular disease[53,54].

In addition to changes in serum IGF-1 and IGFBPs, IGF-1 action may be altered by changes in receptor expression. In skeletal muscle and adipose tissue, the expression of insulin/IGF hybrid receptors is increased in type 2 diabetes and primary hyperinsulinaemia, whilst insulin receptor numbers fall[55,56]. Muscle is the principal site of insulin-stimulated glucose disposal *in vivo*, with less glucose being transported into adipose tissue. A fall in IGF-1 may result in reduced insulin-like activity in tissues expressing high levels of IGF-1 receptors, such as muscle. Glucose uptake in these cells would be impaired and glucose would be taken up preferentially by cells which do not express IGF receptors, such as adipocytes. This phenomenon may be exacerbated in states of hyperinsulinaemia as occurs with insulin resistance. A metabolic consequence of this scenario would be enhanced insulin-mediated lipogenesis in adipocytes at the expense of reduced muscle glycogen synthesis.

There is evidence that differential insulin resistance in separate tissues may cause different phenotypes. Specifically, knocking out the insulin receptor in muscle or fat has produced unexpected and informative findings. The muscle insulin receptor knockout mouse has a phenotype, which is similar to the metabolic syndrome[57]. The animals are centrally obese and have dyslipidaemia despite normal glucose tolerance. In contrast, fat insulin receptor knockout mice remain thin despite an unrestricted diet and have normal circulating lipids[58]. It is conceivable that reduced 'insulin-like' action in muscle through reduced IGF-1 may result in a similar phenotype to the muscle insulin receptor knockout mouse.

Regulation of GH–IGF

Growth hormone (GH) exerts its actions through specific cell surface receptors[59]. Although GH has both metabolic and anabolic actions, most of its anabolic actions are mediated through the generation of IGF-1[60]. IGF-1 has profound anabolic and metabolic effects in many cell types, acting through autocrine, paracrine and classical endocrine mechanisms[61]. IGF-1 has major insulin-like effects on many cell types expressing the IGF-1 receptor, including skeletal muscle, where it stimulates glucose uptake, glycolysis and glycogen synthesis. On a molar basis, there is about 250–1000 times more IGF-1 in the circulation than insulin. However, less than 5% is free, with 90% bound in a stable ternary complex comprising IGF-1, IGFBP-3 and an acid labile subunit[62]. The remaining IGF-1 is bound by IGFBP-1, IGFBP-2 or IGFBP-4[63,64]. Despite free IGF-1 having only ~10% of the effect of insulin on glucose metabolism[65], its excess ensures that it contributes significantly to insulin-like activity.

IGF-1 is present in the circulation and throughout the extracellular space almost entirely bound to members of a family of at least six high affinity IGF binding proteins (IGFBP-1 to IGFBP-6)[61]. The IGFBPs are essential to co-ordinate and regulate the biological functions of the IGFs. Within the circulation, they transport IGFs and control their efflux from the circulation. IGF-1 exerts its actions primarily through the IGF-1 receptor[66]. IGF-1 may also bind to the insulin receptor. However, IGR-1 affinity for the insulin receptor is approximately 1% that of insulin[67]. Hybrid receptors, containing halves of the insulin and IGF receptor, occur widely in mammalian tissues. Their physiological significance remains unclear but they bind IGF-1 more readily than insulin[68]. The differential, receptor-mediated actions of IGF-1 and insulin may relate to the relative affinities of ligands for their respective receptors and the distribution of the receptors. Insulin receptors predominate in hepatocytes and adipocytes, while IGF-1 receptors are expressed mainly in mesenchymal cells, such as fibroblasts and myocytes[69]. Therefore, the actions of IGF-1 in muscle may be particularly important in up-regulating muscle insulin sensitivity.

Epidemiological studies have shown an association between low levels of physical activity, fitness and the metabolic syndrome[70]. Conversely, exercise has a beneficial effect on body composition, with increased muscle bulk and reduced fat mass, in both normal and GH-deficient adults. In some patients with GH deficiency, the benefits of exercise may exceed those seen with conventional GH replacement therapy. These improvements may be mediated, in part, by increases in both circulating and locally produced IGF-1 in muscle. Circulating IGF-1 correlates with fitness and training in young rats while exercise causes an increase in IGF-1 stimulated protein synthesis in muscle[71]. Exercise may improve insulin sensitivity by increasing paracrine and autocrine IGF-1 mediated glucose uptake by muscle, possibly by increasing GLUT-4 content[72] or by increasing GH levels.

The early environment and GH–IGF action

Poor intra-uterine growth may affect the GH–IGF axis. Studies in humans suggest that low birth weight is associated with a number of abnormalities in the GH–IGF axis, which affect GH secretion and action and there also seems to be important interactions occurring between the GH–IGF axis and the effects of adult obesity. Individuals in the highest birth weight group (> 3600 g) who remained non-obese in adult life (BMI < 22 kg/m^2) had a mean urinary GH excretion almost 5 times higher than subjects in the lowest birth weight group (< 3200 g) who were overweight in adult life (BMI > 26 kg/m^2). Urinary GH levels, which reflect GH secretion, are low in young adults of low birth weight[73]. Prenatal and early postnatal studies have shown that poor fetal growth is associated with GH resistance, which is characterised by high serum GH and low IGF-1 levels[74]. There are also abnormalities in serum IGFBPs, resulting in high IGFBP-1 and IGFBP-2 and low IGFBP-3 levels[75]. The interactions between IGF-1 and its binding proteins are complex and it is difficult to predict the change in IGF-1 bioactivity *in vivo* as a result of alterations in serum IGFBPs. However, it could be expected that the combined changes in IGFBP-1 to IGFBP-3 would be inhibitory on the action of IGF-1.

Most studies have shown that poor intra-uterine nutrition results in a lower plasma IGF-1 in umbilical cord blood compared to babies of the same gestational age who are well nourished. Fetal plasma glucose and insulin concentrations are major determinants of the fetal IGF secretion, so reduced fetal plasma glucose and insulin concentrations as a result of maternal undernutrition may explain the fall in fetal plasma IGF-1. GH secretion is pulsatile in pre- and postnatal life and pulses are the result of a balance between the stimulatory action of GH releasing hormone and the inhibitory action of somatostatin. It has been shown in sheep that undernutrition has no effect on GH pulsatility, but there may be reduction in inhibition of endogenous GHRH in response to GH[76]. Moreover, undernutrition may influence somatostatin levels and, therefore, the

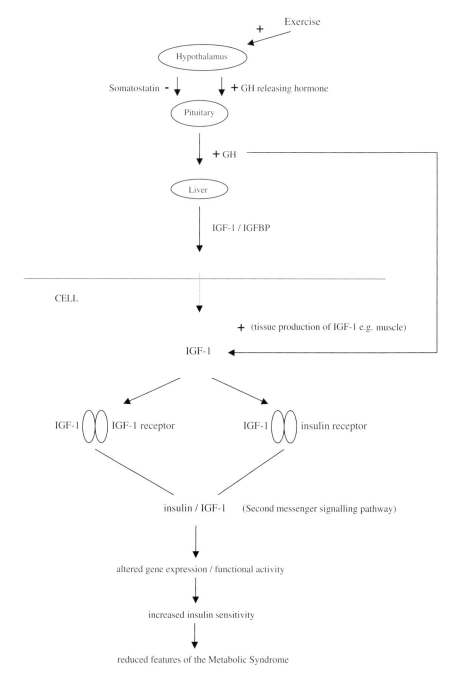

Fig. 4 Schematic representation of the growth hormone–insulin like growth factor axis and insulin like growth factor action.

inhibition of GH levels. A 50% reduction in fetal GH concentration has been demonstrated during an infusion of somatostatin in fetal lambs[76] and an *in vitro* study has shown dose-dependent inhibition of GH by somatostatin from mid-gestation onward, in human pituitary cells[77].

Maternal dietary restriction during gestation and lactation causes persisting reductions in GH secretion in the offspring[78,79]. Low birth weight babies have high basal GH but low IGF-1 concentrations at birth[80,81] with an increased GH response to growth hormone releasing hormone[82]. In childhood, low birth weight is associated with a high baseline secretion of GH but low amplitude peaks[83,84]. The only study in adult life is an analysis of GH secretory profile in 37 men, aged 63–73 years which showed no relationship with birth weight but found that low infant weight was associated with reduced median GH secretion[85].

Thus, in summary, the available evidence supports the notion that low birth weight and adult obesity are associated with reduced levels of IGF-1. From the evidence presented above, this suggests a mechanism linking low birth weight and adult obesity with insulin resistance (particularly in muscle) and the metabolic syndrome. Low growth rates *in utero* may programme abnormalities of the GH-IGF axis resulting in decreased IGF-1 activity. A schematic representation is shown in Figure 4, illustrating regulation of the GH–IGF axis and IGF action and development of the metabolic syndrome.

Conclusions

Low birth weight is associated with type 2 diabetes and AVD in adulthood. The evidence suggests that type 2 diabetes and AVD share a common aetiology mediated by insulin resistance and other features of the metabolic syndrome. Since reduced early growth and subsequent adult central obesity markedly increases risk of the metabolic syndrome in adulthood, reduced early growth may contribute to type 2 diabetes and AVD in adulthood by predisposing to the metabolic syndrome. Increased glucocorticoid hormone action and reduced IGF-1 activity contribute to development of the metabolic syndrome and may mediate a link between low birth weight, adult obesity, type 2 diabetes and AVD.

Acknowledgements

I thank Professor DI Phillips, Dr RI Holt, Dr CB Whorwood and Dr J Zhang for their contributions, Ms C Kyme for her assistance and the MRC for their support.

References

1   Stern MP. Do non-insulin-dependent diabetes mellitus and cardiovascular disease share common antecedents? *Ann Intern Med* 1996; **124**: 110–6

2   Reaven GM. Banting Lecture 1988. Role of insulin resistance in human disease. *Diabetes* 1988; **37**: 1595–607

3   Barker DJP. Fetal origins of coronary heart disease. *BMJ* 1995; **311**: 171–4

4   Hales CN, Barker DJP, Clark PM *et al*. Fetal and infant growth and impaired glucose tolerance at age 64. *BMJ* 1991; **303**: 1019–22

5   Barker DJP, Hales CN, Fall CH, Osmond C, Phipps K, Clark PM. Type 2 (non-insulin-dependent) diabetes mellitus, hypertension and hyperlipidaemia (syndrome X): relation to reduced fetal growth. *Diabetologia* 1993; **36**: 62–7

6   Valdez R, Athens MA, Thompson GH, Bradshaw BS, Stern MP. Birthweight and adult health outcomes in a biethnic population in the USA. *Diabetologia* 1994; **37**: 624–31

7   McKeigue PM, Lithell HO, Leon DA. Glucose tolerance and resistance to insulin-stimulated glucose uptake in men aged 70 years in relation to size at birth. *Diabetologia* 1998; **41**: 1133–8

8   Clausen JO, Borch-Johnsen K, Pederson O. Relation between birthweight and the insulin sensitivity index in a population sample of 331 young healthy Caucasians. *Am J Epidemiol* 1996; **146**: 23–31

9   Phillips DI. Birth weight and the future development of diabetes. A review of the evidence. *Diabetes Care* 1998; **21 (Suppl 2)**: B150–5

10 Lithell HO, McKeigue PM, Berglund L, Mohsen R, Lithell UB, Leon DA. Relation of size at birth to non-insulin dependent diabetes and insulin concentrations in men aged 50–60 years. *BMJ* 1996; **312**: 406–10

11 Orth DN, Kovacs WJ. The adrenal cortex. In: Wilson JD, Foster DW, Kronenberg HM, Larsen PR. (eds) *Williams Textbook of Endocrinology*, 9th edn. New York: WB Saunders, 1998; 517–665

12 Björntorp P. Insulin resistance: the consequence of a neuroendocrine disturbance? *Int J Obes* 1995; **19 (Suppl 1)**: S6–10

13 Pasquali R, Cantobelli S, Casimirri F *et al*. The hypothalamic–pituitary–adrenal axis in obese women with different patterns of body fat distribution. *J Clin Endocrinol Metab* 1993; **77**: 341–6

14 Phillips DI, Barker DJ, Fall CH *et al*. Elevated plasma cortisol concentrations: a link between low birth weight and the insulin resistance syndrome? *J Clin Endocrinol Metab* 1998; **83**: 757–60

15 Stolk RP, Lamberts SW, de Jong FH, Pols HA, Grobbee DE. Gender differences in the associations between cortisol and insulin in healthy subjects. *J Endocrinol* 1996; **149**: 313–8

16 Filipovsky J, Ducimetiére P, Eschwége E, Richard JL, Rosselin G, Claude JR. The relationship of blood pressure with glucose, insulin, heart rate, free fatty acids and plasma cortisol levels according to degree of obesity in middle-aged men. *J Hypertens* 1996; **14**: 229–35

17 Rosmond R, Dallman MF, Björntorp P. Stress-related cortisol secretion in men: relationships with abdominal obesity and endocrine, metabolic and hemodynamic abnormalities. *J Clin Endocrinol Metab* 1998; **83**: 1853–9

18 Mårin P, Darin N, Amemiya T, Andersson B, Jern S, Björntorp P. Cortisol secretion in relation to body fat distribution in obese premenopausal women. *Metabolism* 1992; **41**: 882–6

19 Hautanen A, Adlercreutz H. Altered adrenocorticotropin and cortisol secretion in abdominal obesity: implications for the insulin resistance syndrome. *J Intern Med* 1993; **234**: 461–9

20 Weaver JU, Hitman GA, Kopelman PG. An association between a BclI restriction fragment length polymorphism of the glucocorticoid receptor locus and hyperinsulinaemia in obese women. *J Mol Endocrinol* 1992; **9**: 295–300

21 Kenyon CJ, Panarelli M, Zagato L *et al*. Glucocorticoid receptor polymorphism in genetic hypertension. *J Mol Endocrinol* 1998; **21**: 41–50

22 Panarelli M, Holloway CD, Fraser R *et al*. Glucocorticoid receptor polymorphism, skin vasoconstriction, and other metabolic intermediate phenotypes in normal human subjects. *J Clin Endocrinol Metab* 1998; **83**: 1846–52

23 Buemann B, Vohl MC, Chagnon M *et al*. Abdominal visceral fat is associated with a BclI restriction fragment length polymorphism at the glucocorticoid receptor gene locus. *Obes Res* 1997; **5**: 186–92

24 Hollenberg SM, Weinberger C, Ong ES *et al*. Primary structure and expression of a functional human glucocorticoid receptor cDNA. *Nature* 1985; **318**: 635–41

25 Bamberger CM, Schulte HM, Chrousos GP. Molecular determinants of glucocorticoid receptor function and tissue sensitivity to glucocorticoids. *Endocr Rev* 1996; **17**: 245–61

26 White PC, Mune T, Agarwal AK. 11 beta-hydroxysteroid dehydrogenase and the syndrome of apparent mineralocorticoid excess. *Endocr Rev* 1997; **18**: 135–56

27 Naray-Fejes-Toth A, Colombowala IK, Fejes-Toth G. The role of 11beta-hydroxysteroid dehydrogenase in steroid hormone specificity. *J Steroid Biochem Mol Biol* 1998; **65**: 311–6

28 Whorwood CB, Mason JI, Ricketts ML, Howie AJ, Stewart PM. Detection of human 11 beta-hydroxysteroid dehydrogenase isoforms using reverse-transcriptase-polymerase chain reaction and localization of the type 2 isoform to renal collecting ducts. *Mol Cell Endocrinol* 1995; **110**: R7–12

29 Whorwood CB, Ricketts ML, Stewart PM. Epithelial cell localization of type 2 11 beta-hydroxysteroid dehydrogenase in rat and human colon. *Endocrinology* 1994; **135**: 2533–41

30 Langley-Evans SC. Intrauterine programming of hypertension by glucocorticoids. *Life Sci* 1997; **60**: 1213–21

31 Benediktsson R, Lindsay RS, Noble J, Seckl JR, Edwards CR. Glucocorticoid exposure *in utero*: new model for adult hypertension. *Lancet* 1993; **341**: 339–41

32 Seckl JR. Glucocorticoids and small babies [editorial]. *Q J Med* 1994; **87**: 259–62

33 Tangalakis K, Lumbers ER, Moritz KM, Towstoless MK, Wintour EM. Effect of cortisol on blood pressure and vascular reactivity in the ovine fetus. *Exp Physiol* 1992; **77**: 709–17

34 Goland RS, Jozak S, Warren WB, Conwell IM, Stark RI, Tropper PJ. Elevated levels of umbilical cord plasma corticotropin-releasing hormone in growth-retarded fetuses. *J Clin Endocrinol Metab* 1993; **77**: 1174–9

35 Edwards CR, Benediktsson R, Lindsay RS, Seckl JR. Dysfunction of placental glucocorticoid barrier: link between fetal environment and adult hypertension? *Lancet* 1993; **341**: 355–7

36 Walker BR, Phillips DI, Noon JP *et al.* Increased glucocorticoid activity in men with cardiovascular risk factors. *Hypertension* 1998; **31**: 891–5

37 Kotelevtsev Y, Seckl JR, Mullins JJ. Hydroxysteroid dehydrogenases: key modulators of glucocorticoids in vivo. *Curr Opin Endocrinol Diabetes* 1999; **6**: 191–8

38 Zhang J, Desai M, Ozanne SE, Doherty C, Hales CN, Byrne CD. Two variants of quantitative reverse transcriptase PCR used to show differential expression of alpha-, beta- and gamma-fibrinogen genes in rat liver lobes. *Biochem J* 1997; **321**: 769–75

39 Zhang J, Byrne CD. A novel highly reproducible quantitative competitive RT PCR system. *J Mol Biol* 1997; **274**: 338–52

40 Zhang J, Byrne CD. Differential priming of RNA templates during cDNA synthesis markedly affects both accuracy and reproducibility of quantitative competitive reverse-transcriptase PCR. *Biochem J* 1999; **337**: 231–41

41 Barbazanges A, Piazza PV, Le Moal M, Maccari S. Maternal glucocorticoid secretion mediates long-term effects of prenatal stress. *J Neurosci* 1996; **16**: 3943–9

42 Reul JM, Stec I, Wiegers GJ *et al.* Prenatal immune challenge alters the hypothalamic-pituitary-adrenocortical axis in adult rats. *J Clin Invest* 1994; **93**: 2600–7

43 Lee S, Imaki T, Vale W, Rivier C. Effect of prenatal exposure to ethanol on the activity of the hypothalamic–pituitary–adrenal axis' activity of the offspring: importance of the time of exposure to ethanol and possible modulating mechanisms. *Mol Cell Neurosci* 1990; **1**: 168–77

44 Lindsay RS, Lindsay RM, Edwards CR, Seckl JR. Inhibition of 11β hydroxysteroid dehydrogenase in pregnant rats and the programming of blood pressure in the offspring. *Hypertension* 1996; **27**: 1200–4

45 Levitt NS, Lindsay RS, Holmes MC, Seckl JR. Dexamethasone in the last week of pregnancy attenuates hippocampal glucocorticoid receptor gene expression and elevates blood pressure in the adult offspring in the rat. *Neuroendocrinology* 1996; **64**: 412–8

46 Saitoh H, Kamoda T, Nakahara S, Hirano T, Nakamura N. Serum concentrations of insulin, insulin-like growth factor(IGF)-I, IGF binding protein (IGFBP)-1 and -3 and growth hormone binding protein in obese children: fasting IGFBP-1 is suppressed in normoinsulinaemic obese children. *Clin Endocrinol* 1998; **48**: 487–92

47 Ceda GP, Dall'Aglio E, Magnacavallo A *et al.* The insulin-like growth factor axis and plasma lipid levels in the elderly. *J Clin Endocrinol Metab* 1998; **83**: 499–502

48 Gibson JM, Westwood M, Young RJ, White A. Reduced insulin-like growth factor binding

protein-1 (IGFBP-1) levels correlate with increased cardiovascular risk in non-insulin dependent diabetes mellitus (NIDDM). *J Clin Endocrinol Metab* 1996; **81**: 860–3

49 Sartorio A, Conti A, Ferrero S. Low urinary GH levels in normal statured obese children. *Acta Paediatr* 1996; **85**: 894–8

50 Veldhuis JD, Iranmanesh A, Ho KK, Waters MJ, Johnson ML, Lizarralde G. Dual defects in pulsatile growth hormone secretion and clearance subserve the hyposomatotropism of obesity in man. *J Clin Endocrinol Metab* 1991; **72**: 51–9

51 Björntorp P. The origins and consequences of obesity. *Diabetes* 1996; **201**: 68–80; discussion 80–9, 188–93

52 Saccà L, Cittadini A, Fazio S. Growth hormone and the heart. *Endocr Rev* 1994; **15**: 555–73

53 Rosén T, Bengtsson BA. Premature mortality due to cardiovascular disease in hypopituitarism. *Lancet* 1990; **336**: 285–8

54 Maison P, Balkau B, Simon D, Chanson P, Rosselin G, Eschwège E. Growth hormone as a risk for premature mortality in healthy subjects: data from the Paris prospective study. *BMJ* 1998; **316**: 1132–3

55 Federici M, Lauro D, D'Adamo M *et al*. Expression of insulin/IGF-1 hybrid receptors is increased in skeletal muscle of patients with chronic primary hyperinsulinemia. *Diabetes* 1998; **47**: 87–92

56 Federici M, Porzio O, Zucaro L *et al*. Increased abundance of insulin/IGF-1 hybrid receptors in adipose tissue from NIDDM patients. *Mol Cell Endocrinol* 1997; **135**: 41–7

57 Bruning JC, Michael MD, Winnay JN *et al*. A muscle-specific insulin receptor knockout exhibits features of the metabolic syndrome of NIDDM without altering glucose tolerance. *Mol Cell* 1998; **2**: 559–69

58 Kahn CR, Iacocca MK. Knockout mice challenge our concepts of glucose, homeostasis and the pathogenesis of diabetes. *The Endocrine Society's 81st Annual Meeting*, 1999; L6, P 17

59 Leung DW, Spencer SA, Cachianes G *et al*. Growth hormone receptor and serum binding protein: purification, cloning and expression. *Nature* 1987; **330**: 537–43

60 Mathews LS, Hammer RE, Brinster RL, Palmiter RD. Expression of insulin-like growth factor I in transgenic mice with elevated levels of growth hormone is correlated with growth. *Endocrinology* 1988; **123**: 433–7

61 Jones JI, Clemmons DR. Insulin-like growth factors and their binding proteins: biological actions. *Endocr Rev* 1995; **16**: 3–34

62 Martin JL, Baxter RC. Insulin-like growth factor binding protein-3: biochemistry and physiology. *Growth Regul* 1992; **2**: 88–99

63 Zapf J, Kiefer M, Merryweather J *et al*. Isolation from adult human serum of four insulin-like growth factor (IGF) binding proteins and molecular cloning of one of them that is increased by IGF 1 administration and in extrapancreatic tumor hypoglycemia. *J Biol Chem* 1990; **265**: 14892–8

64 Kiefer MC, Masiarz FR, Bauer DM, Zapf J. Identification and molecular cloning of two new 30-kDa insulin-like growth factor binding proteins isolated from adult human serum. *J Biol Chem* 1991; **266**: 9043–9

65 Russell-Jones DL, Bates AT, Umpleby AM *et al*. A comparison of the effects of IGF-1 and insulin on glucose metabolism, fat metabolism and the cardiovascular system in normal human volunteers. *Eur J Clin Invest* 1995; **25**: 403–11

66 Jacobs S, Kull FCJ, Earp HS, Svoboda ME, Van Wyk JJ, Cuatrecasas P. Somatomedin-C stimulates the phosphorylation of the beta-subunit of its own receptor. *J Biol Chem* 1983; **258**: 9581–4

67 Czech MP. Signal transmission by the insulin-like growth factors. *Cell* 1989; **59**: 235–8

68 Siddle K, Soos MA, Field CE, Nave BT. Hybrid and atypical insulin/insulin-like growth factor I receptors. *Horm Res* 1994; **41**: 56–64

69 Froesch ER, Zapf J. Insulin-like growth factors and insulin: comparative aspects. *Diabetologia* 1985; **28**: 485–93

70 Wareham NJ, Hennings SJ, Byrne CD, Hales CN, Prentice AM, Day NE. A quantitative analysis of the relationship between habitual energy expenditure, fitness and the metabolic cardiovascular syndrome. *Br J Nutr* 1998; **80**: 235–41

71 Eliakim A, Moromisato M, Moromisato D, Brasel JA, Roberts CJ, Cooper DM. Increase in

muscle IGF-1 protein but not IGF-1 mRNA after 5 days of endurance training in young rats. *Am J Physiol* 1997; **273**: R1557–61

72   Willis PE, Chadan SG, Baracos V, Parkhouse WS. Restoration of insulin-like growth factor I action in skeletal muscle of old mice. *Am J Physiol* 1998; **275**: E525–30

73   Flanagan DE, Moore VM, Godsland IF, Cockington RA, Robinson JS, Phillips DI. Reduced foetal growth and growth hormone secretion in adult life. *Clin Endocrinol* 1999; **50**: 735–40

74   Cianfarani S, Germani D, Rossi P *et al*. Intrauterine growth retardation: evidence for the activation of the insulin-like growth factor (IGF) – related growth-promoting machinery and the presence of a cation-independent IGF binding protein-3 proteolytic activity by two months of life. *Pediatr Res* 1998; **44**: 374–80

75   Langford K, Blum W, Nicolaides K, Jones J, McGregor A, Miell J. The pathophysiology of the insulin-like growth factor axis in fetal growth failure: a basis for programming by undernutrition? *Eur J Clin Invest* 1994; **24**: 851–6

76   Bauer MK, Breier BH, Harding JE, Veldhuis JD, Gluckman PD. The fetal somatotropic axis during long term maternal undernutrition in sheep; evidence for nutritional regulation in utero. *Endocrinology* 1994; **136**: 1250–7

77   Goodyer CG, Branchaud CL, Lefebvre Y. Effects of growth hormone (GH)-releasing factor and somatostatin on GH secretion from early to mid-gestation human fetal pituitaries. *J Clin Endocrinol Metab* 1993; **76**: 1259–64

78   Stephan JK, Chow B, Frohman LA, Chow BF. Relationship of growth hormone to the growth retardation associated with maternal dietary restriction. *J Nutr* 1971; **101**: 1453–8

79   Harel Z, Tannenbaum GS. Long-term alterations in growth hormone and insulin secretion after temporary dietary protein restriction in early life in the rat. *Pediatr Res* 1995; **38**: 747–53

80   de Zegher F, Kimpen J, Raus J, Vanderschueren-Lodeweyckx M. Hypersomatotropism in the dysmature infant at term and preterm birth. *Biol Neonate* 1990; **58**: 188–91

81   Ackland FM, Stanhope R, Eyre C, Hamill G, Jones J, Preece MA. Physiological growth hormone secretion in children with short stature and intra-uterine growth retardation. *Horm Res* 1988; **30**: 241–5

82   Deiber M, Chatelain P, Naville D, Putet G, Salle B. Functional hypersomatotropism in small for gestational age (SGA) newborn infants. *J Clin Endocrinol Metab* 1989; **68**: 232–4

83   Albertsson-Wikland K. Growth hormone secretion and growth hormone treatment in children with intrauterine growth retardation. Swedish Paediatric Study Group for Growth Hormone Treatment. *Acta Paediatr Scand Suppl* 1989; **349**: 35–41; discussion 53–4

84   Boguszewski M, Rosberg S, Albertsson-Wikland K. Spontaneous 24-hour growth hormone profiles in prepubertal small for gestational age children. *J Clin Endocrinol Metab* 1995; **80**: 2599–606

85   Fall C, Hindmarsh P, Dennison E, Kellingray S, Barker D, Cooper C. Programming of growth hormone secretion and bone mineral density in elderly men: a hypothesis. *J Clin Endocrinol Metab* 1998; **83**: 135–9

Long-term consequences for offspring of diabetes during pregnancy

Frans A Van Assche, Kathleen Holemans and **Leona Aerts**

Department of Obstetrics and Gynaecology, University Hospital Gasthuisberg, Leuven, Belgium

There is evidence that the diabetic intra-uterine environment has consequences for later life. Maternal diabetes mainly results in asymmetric macrosomia. This macrosomia is associated with an increased insulin secretion and overstimulation of the insulin producing B-cells during fetal life. In later life, a reduced insulin secretion is found. Intra-uterine growth restriction is present in severe maternal diabetes associated with vasculopathy. Intra-uterine growth restriction is associated with low insulin secretion and reduced development of the insulin receptors. In later life, these alterations can induce insulin resistance. The long-term consequences of an abnormal intra-uterine environment are of primary importance world-wide. Concentrated efforts are needed to explore how these long-term effects can be prevented.

Fetal growth and development are partly determined by the fetal genome, but the genetic regulation of fetal growth is influenced by different factors, which can exert a stimulatory or an inhibitory effect. Fetal growth is dependent on the capacity of the mother to supply nutrients and also on the capacity of the placenta to transfer these nutrients to the fetus. But the fetus has its own growth factors which influence growth and differentiation. Normal fetal growth depends on an equilibrium in the interaction between these different compartments and between stimulatory and inhibitory factors. When this equilibrium is disturbed, intra-uterine growth restriction (microsomia) or fetal overgrowth (macrosomia) can be the consequence[1]. Both abnormalities in fetal growth are related to an abnormal intra-uterine environment.

In the human, fetal macrosomia is the most important finding in maternal diabetes, since there is increased supply of glucose and other nutrients[2,3]. However, in severe maternal diabetes complicated by vasculopathy and nephropathy, intra-uterine growth restriction can be present[4].

The present review will first concentrate on human fetal development and fetal growth in a diabetic intra-uterine environment and discuss the consequences for these offspring in later life. Second, we will briefly explore the working mechanisms in an experimental design in animal studies on diabetes and pregnancy.

Correspondence to:
Prof. Dr F A Van Assche,
Department of Obstetrics
and Gynaecology,
University Hospital
Gasthuisberg,
Herestraat 49,
B-3000 Leuven, Belgium

Fetal development and fetal growth in a diabetic intra-uterine environment and the consequences for later life in the human

Maternal diabetes is characterised by an increased placental transport of glucose and other nutrients from the mother to the fetus, resulting in macrosomia[2,3]. In the endocrine pancreas islet hypertrophy and hyperplasia of the insulin producing B-cells have been recognised for many years as typical features in fetuses and newborn babies of diabetic mothers[5-11]. The features of B-cell stimulation are observed as early as 19 weeks of gestation[12]. An increased insulin secretion coincides with an increased amount of insulin producing B-cells (see Fowden & Hill, this issue). Simultaneously, levels of insulin-like growth factors (IGF) also increase. Both insulin and IGFs are related to birth weight[13].

Macrosomia can be divided into a symmetric and asymmetric type. Symmetric fetal overgrowth may be due to genetic factors, whereas asymmetric fetal overgrowth is induced in a diabetic intra-uterine environment with an increased maternal–fetal nutrient transfer. This macrosomia is characterised by an enlarged thoracic and abdominal circumference, which is relatively larger than the head circumference.

We have recently shown that features of B-cell hyperplasia and of hyperinsulinism are only present in macrosomic fetuses of the asymmetric type and not in macrosomic fetuses of the symmetric type[14]. Infiltration by eosinophilic polymorphs in and around the fetal islets is only present in type I diabetes[15].

Insulin is stored in typical granules in B-cells. In situations of excessive stimulation of the B-cells, the stores are used for secretion. Degranulation of the B-cells is, therefore, seen as an expression of overstimulation. In a newborn of a badly controlled diabetic mother (blood glucose >16.7 mmol/l), we found degranulated B-cells with swollen mitochondria, extended rough endoplasmic recticulum and very few granules, as described in fetuses of severely diabetic rats[16].

The study of anencephalics also provides interesting data. The basal development of the fetal endocrine pancreas is normal; however, B-cell hyperplasia and increased insulin secretion is only present in anencephalics with a functional hypothalamic-hypophyseal (HH) system born to diabetic mothers. Furthermore, only these anencephalics are macrosomic[11]. A summary of the morphometric data is presented in Table 1.

In severe maternal diabetes associated with vasculopathy and reduced renal function, intra-uterine growth restriction may be present; we have shown that insulin secretion and the number of B-cells are reduced[17]. It may be stressed that fetal development in a diabetic environment is characterised by an increased insulin secretion, due to overstimulation and possibly resulting in exhaustion of the fetal pancreatic B-cells. These

Table I Morphometric data of the human fetal endocrine pancreas (mean ± SD)

	Volume density of endocrine tissue	Percentage of B cells
Normal controls (n = 40)	5.1 ± 1.6	40 ± 7.5
Maternal diabetes (n = 10)	12.9 ± 4.2	63.8 ± 8.9
Anencephalics without a functional HH system of a diabetic mother (n = 8)	5.0 ± 1.6	38 ± 9.7
Anencephalics with a functional HH system of a diabetic mother (n = 7)	11.6 ± 4.9	59.2 ± 6.9

alterations in fetal life may explain the consequences in later life. Degranulation of the fetal insulin producing B-cells can be found when extremely high glucose levels in the mother are present[16].

The risk for diabetes is significantly higher when the mother rather than the father had non-insulin dependent diabetes[18]. Furthermore, 35% of patients with gestational diabetes are offspring of diabetic mothers compared with only 5% of normoglycaemic mothers, and gestational diabetes occurs more frequently in the offspring of diabetic mothers (35%) than in offspring of diabetic fathers (7%)[19]. Most convincing are the studies on Pima Indians which have shown that, besides a genetic transmission of diabetes, the diabetic intra-uterine milieu can also induce a diabetogenic tendency in the offspring. Impaired glucose tolerance is more frequent in children of mothers who had diabetes during pregnancy than in children of mothers who developed diabetes after pregnancy (33% *versus* 14% at age 15–19 years)[20].

However, there is at this time no clear-cut explanation why children of diabetic fathers have a greater risk for type I diabetes than children of pregestational diabetic mothers[21]. The eosinophilic infiltration in islets of newborn babies from diabetic mothers could be a protective mechanism for the development of diabetes, since this infiltration is only seen in infants of type I diabetic mothers and not of mothers with gestational diabetes[22].

An extensive study over several generations demonstrated a predominance of type II diabetes in great-grandmothers of infantile onset diabetes on the maternal side compared with the paternal side. In addition, a predominance of familial diabetes aggregation in first- and second-degree relatives was found on the maternal side compared with the paternal side. Systematic prevention of hyperglycaemia and impaired glucose tolerance in pregnant women has significantly decreased the prevalence of diabetes mellitus in their children[23,24].

As indicated before, asymmetric macrosomia is associated with increased fetal insulin and IGF levels. IGF and insulin have mitogenic effects on the fetal breast tissue. This may explain the increased incidence of breast carcinoma in women who where macrosomic at birth[25].

Intra-uterine growth restriction can be present in severe maternal diabetes complicated by vasculopathy. The perinatal mortality in these growth retarded newborn babies of diabetic mothers has been high, and little information is available on the long-term consequences.

Animal models

Mild maternal diabetes

When the mother has mild diabetes (glycaemia increased by ± 20%) during pregnancy, induced by destroying part of the B-cells[26,27] or by continuous glucose infusion[28], increased amounts of glucose reach the fetus by facilitated transfer through the placenta. In order to deal with this abundant glucose supply, adaptations occur in fetal insulin production and insulin action. The development of the fetal islets of Langerhans is enhanced, resulting in hypertrophy of the endocrine pancreas and hyperplasia of the B-cells. Not only the number of fetal B-cells is increased, but also the biosynthetic activity of the individual insulin producing cell is enhanced[26]. The insulin response to glucose stimulation, both *in vivo* and *in vitro*, is clearly increased in the fetuses of mildly diabetic mothers as compared to controls[27].

After withdrawal of the hyperglycaemic maternal stimulus at birth, the lactation period appears to represent a poor stimulus for the further development of the endocrine pancreas, which ends up hypoplastic by the time of weaning[26]. However, at adulthood, the offspring of mildly diabetic mothers display a normal mass of endocrine pancreas, with a normal contribution of the different islet-cell types[29]. Glycaemia and insulinaemia are normal, at least in basal conditions. On glucose stimulation, however, *in vivo* and *in vitro* insulin response is deficient. In this and other experiments with perinatal hyperinsulinaemia[25,28,30–32], glucose tolerance in the adult animal is impaired.

Severe maternal diabetes

When maternal rats are made severely diabetic (by destroying the majority of their B-cells), the fetuses are confronted with very high glucose concentrations. The severe fetal hyperglycaemia induces islet hypertrophy and B-cell hyperactivity, and may result in early hyperinsulinaemia. This adaptation, however, appears to be limited, B-cells are overstimulated and the secretion of insulin is faster than its biosynthesis. B-cells become depleted of insulin and often appear disorganized and almost depleted of insulin granules[26]. These degranulated cells are incapable of insulin secretion *in vivo* and *in vitro*[27] and B-cell exhaustion results in fetal hypoinsulinaemia. Hypoinsulinaemia and a reduced number of insulin receptors on target cells[32] lead to a reduction in fetal glucose uptake[33]. The growth of fetal protein mass is suppressed and fetal protein synthesis is consistently lower than in controls[34]. Circulating amino acid levels in the fetuses of severely diabetic mothers are lower than in the controls; the fetal levels parallel the low maternal levels and the feto-maternal ratio is normal[35]. Taurine levels, however, are exceptionally low in mothers and fetuses.

Postnatal development of the microsomic pups born to severely diabetic mothers is retarded, and the animals remain small up to adulthood[26]. At adult age, the endocrine pancreatic mass in these animals exceeds control values, and this excess of islet mass is due to a high number of very small islets of Langerhans[29], suggesting an increased contribution of B-cell neogenesis, rather than cell replication.

Plasma amino acid concentrations are normal in the adult offspring of severely diabetic mothers, including the levels for the neurotransmitters taurine, GABA and carnosine[35]. *In vivo* and *in vitro* stimulation of B-cells exerts an increased secretion of insulin[26].

Furthermore, these offspring are markedly resistant to the action of insulin as revealed by the euglycaemic hyperinsulinaemic clamp[36,37]. The decreased sensitivity to insulin is observed in the liver as well as the extrahepatic tissues[36] and peripheral glucose uptake is specifically reduced in skeletal muscles[37]. The insulin resistance can partly, but not completely, be restored by normalizing maternal glycaemia with islet transplantation in the course of, or even before, pregnancy[38,39]. Insulin sensitivity in any tissue is dependent not only on the ability of insulin to stimulate cellular glucose uptake, but is also influenced by the arteriovenous glucose gradient and, potentially, blood flow[40,41]. Therefore, we determined cardiovascular function, *i.e.* blood pressure, heart rate and vascular function, in the offspring of severely diabetic rats[42]. Exposure to severe maternal diabetes during fetal and neonatal life has profound consequences for cardiovascular function in the offspring. Despite normal systolic and diastolic blood pressure, there is evidence of pronounced bradycardia. The offspring of severely diabetic rats also show abnormalities of vascular function *in vitro*. Mesenteric arteries isolated from adult offspring of diabetic rats show a reduced relaxation to endothelium-dependent dilators and enhanced constriction to noradrenaline. The enhanced sensitivity, but similar maximal response, to noradrenaline is indicative of abnormal receptor-mediated tension development.

The reduction in relaxation to acetylcholine and bradykinin is suggestive of impaired synthesis of endothelium-derived vasodilators. The defect in sensitivity and maximal relaxation to acetylcholine is not observed in the presence of cyclooxygenase, nitric oxide synthase and guanylate synthase blockade, suggesting that prostacyclin/nitric oxide-induced relaxation is responsible for the defect in endothelium-dependent relaxation in offspring of severely diabetic rats, and not an endothelium derived hyperpolarizing factor[42]. The normal sensitivity to sodium nitroprusside also suggests that the defect does not arise from reduced sensitivity of the smooth muscle to nitric oxide, but from reduced nitric oxide synthesis.

Endothelial dysfunction, similar to that we reported in offspring of diabetic rats, is not only observed in adult diabetic subjects[43] and animals[44], but in other conditions with high cardiovascular risk, particularly hyper-cholesterolaemia[45,46]. It is possible, therefore, that the intra-uterine diabetic milieu has conferred upon the offspring of diabetic rats a predisposition to severe cardiovascular disorders in later life.

Offspring during pregnancy

In the experimental model, it was also possible to obtain information on the transmission of the diabetogenic effect to the next generation. Female offspring of mildly diabetic mothers have increased glucose levels when pregnant. This 'gestational diabetes' induces typical features in their fetuses: macrosomia, islet hypertrophy and hyperinsulinism. When the offspring become adult, they display an impaired glucose tolerance with the same characteristics as offspring of mildly diabetic mothers[26,28,31]. When pregnant, the offspring of severely diabetic rats develop signs of glucose intolerance, they have higher glucose and lower insulin levels than normal pregnant rats. These pregnant offspring do not show the normal pregnancy-induced insulin resistance in the second half of pregnancy[47]. Furthermore, vascular dysfunction shows only a slight deterioration during pregnancy[48]. Interestingly, the plasma concentration of the lipid peroxide 8-epi prostaglandin $F_{2\alpha}$ in pregnant offspring of diabetic rats was also raised above that of the pregnant offspring of control rats[48]. Previously, we have shown that these pregnant offspring of severely diabetic rats develop mild hyperglycaemia[47], which could contribute directly to enhanced free radical synthesis and lipid peroxidation[49]. Pregnancy seems to confer additional 'stress' and so unmask an already compromised balance between free radical synthesis and antioxidant status. We suggest that oxidative stress in the diabetic pregnant rat and her pregnant offspring could potentially play a role in fetal 'programming' and the transmission of a diabetogenic tendency to the next generation through permanent alteration of DNA and tissue damage in the developing fetus.

Conclusions

In 1979, we published the first report on the long-term consequences of an abnormal intra-uterine environment under the title: *Is gestational diabetes an acquired condition*[50]. At that time, we were aware of major scepticism that an abnormal intra-uterine environment could induce consequences in later life. However, 43 cycles of cell division occur between fertilisation and birth, but only 5 occur after birth. This may explain the crucial role of fetal life.

The consequences are mostly seen at older age, since the vitality of the organism is reduced and can no longer compensate for these alterations. Alterations can also be seen at periods in life when increased stimulation is present, such as puberty and pregnancy.

It is clear that epidemiological data are important to demonstrate the importance of the long-term effects in the human situation[51,52]; experimental data can be a guide to explain the working mechanisms.

The maternally-derived changes in fetal plasma composition (glucose, amino acids, fatty acids) certainly influence the development and function of the fetal endocrine pancreas, but they may affect other organs and functions as well, in a direct or an indirect way. High glucose concentrations are know to promote B-cell replication, but the typical B-cell hyperplasia in fetuses of diabetic mothers only occurs if the fetus has a functioning hypothalamo-hypophyseal system[11], stressing the involvement of the derived hormones. Moreover, fetal hyperglycaemia induces fetal hyperinsulinaemia, which is known to damage the ventromedial part of the hypothalamus, controlling insulin secretion by modulating the tone on the nervus vagus[32]; other body functions might be affected as well by similar mechanisms.

Fetal hypoinsulinaemia, resulting from B-cell exhaustion (severe diabetes) or from malnutrition, might have an opposite effect: moreover, it presents a lack of stimulus for the development of the insulin receptor system and this effect may differ between the different insulin-sensitive organs. Fetal responses depend on the metabolic condition of the mother: severe diabetes is associated with hyperglycaemia whereas malnutrition is associated with hypoglycaemia. The metabolic condition of the mother also influences the maturation of the fetal gastrointestinal tract and the extension of the vascularisation, not only in the endocrine pancreas but in several other organs, including the brain[53].

In conclusion, the development of the organs and functions associated with fetal glucose metabolism are determined by the intra-uterine metabolic environment, and the nature of this influence is complex, involving many different aspects and interactions.

The next step in our research needs to explore the prevention of these long-term consequences. Optimal diabetic control, good antenatal and perinatal care for all women in all parts of the world and adequate lactation and nutrition after birth are priorities.

In animal research, it is necessary to develop a stable model of maternal diabetes comparable with the human situation. In human studies, we need to explore gene–early environmental interactions[54]. Studies of the offspring of diabetic mothers have provided unequivocal evidence that alterations in the nutritional environment *in utero* lead to chronic disease in the offspring.

References

1   Aerts L, Holemans K, Van Assche FA. Maternal diabetes during pregnancy: consequences for the offspring. *Diabetes Metab Rev* 1990; **6**: 147

2   Freinkel N. Banting Lecture. Of pregnancy and progeny. *Diabetes* 1980; **29**: 1023–35

3   Pedersen J. *The Pregnant Diabetic and Her Newborn. Problems and Management*, 2nd edn. Baltimore, MD: Williams and Wilkins, 1977

4   Van Assche FA, Holemans K, Aerts L. Fetal growth and consequences for later life. *J Perinat Med* 1998; **26**: 337–46

5   Cardell BS. Hypertrophy and hyperplasia of the pancreatic islets in newborn infants. *J Pathol Bacteriol* 1953; **66**: 335

6   D'Agostino AN, Bahn RC. A histopathology study of the pancreas of infants of diabetic mothers. *Diabetes* 1963; **121**: 327

7   Dubreuil G, Anderodias J. Ilôts de Langerhans géants chez un nouveau-né issue de mère glucosurique. *Comptes Rendus des Séances Sociologiques et Biologiques* 1920; **24**: 1940

8. Jackson WPU, Woolf N. Maternal prediabetes as a cause of unexplained stillbirth. *Diabetes* 1958; **7**: 446

9   Miller HC. Effect of diabetic and prediabetic pregnancy on fetuses and newborn infants. *Pediatrics* 1946; **19**: 445

10 Naeye RL. Infants of diabetic mothers: quantitative morphologic study. *Pediatrics* 1965; **35**: 980–9

11. Van Assche FA. *The Fetal Endocrine Pancreas: A Quantitative Morphological Approach*. PhD thesis, University of Leuven 1970

12 Van Assche FA, Gepts W, Aerts L. The fetal endocrine pancreas in diabetes (human). *Diabetologia* 1976; **12**: 423

13 Verhaeghe J, Van Bree R, Van Herck E, Laureys J, Bouillon R, Van Assche FA. C-peptide, insulin-like growth factors I and II, and insulin-like growth factor binding protein-I and II, and insulin-like growth factor binding protein-I in umbilical cord serum: correlations with birth weight. *Am J Obstet Gynecol* 1993; **169**: 89

14 Van Assche FA. Symmetric and asymmetric fetal macrosomia in relation to long-term consequences. *Am J Obstet Gynecol* 1997; **177**: 1563

15 Van Assche FA, Aerts L, Gepts W. The different cell types in the endocrine pancreas (human). *Diabetologia* 1982; **16**: 151–2

16 Van Assche FA, Aerts L, De Prins FA. Degranulation of the insulin-producing B cells in an infant of a diabetic mother. Case report. *Br J Obstet Gynaecol* 1983; **90**: 182–5

17 Van Assche FA, De Prins F, Aerts L, Verjans M. The endocrine pancreas in small for date infants. *Br J Obstet Gynaecol* 1977; **84**: 751

18 Knowler W, Pettitt DJ, Kunzelman CL, Everhart J. Genetic and environment determinants of non-insulin dependent diabetes mellitus. *Diabetes Res Clin Pract Suppl* 1985; **1**: S309

19 Martin AO, Simpson JL, Ober C, Freinkel N. Frequency of diabetes mellitus in mothers of probands with gestational diabetes: possible maternal influence on the predisposition to gestational diabetes. *Am J Obstet Gynecol* 1985; **151**: 471

20 Pettitt DJ, Aleck KA, Baird HR, Carraher MJ, Bennett PH, Knowler WC. Congenital

susceptibility to NIDDM. Role of intra-uterine environment. *Diabetes* 1988; **37**: 622

21 Warram JH, Martin BC, Krolewski AJ. Possible mechanisms for the diminished risk of IDDM in the children of diabetic mothers. In: Andreani D, Bompiani G, De Maria U, Faulk WP, Galluzo A. (eds) *Immunobiology of Normal and Diabetic Pregnancy*. New York: Wiley, 1990; 221

22 Van Assche FA, Aerts L, Holemans K, Danneels L. Fetal consequences of maternal diabetes. In: Andreani D, Bompiani G, De Maria U, Faulk WP, Galluzo A. (eds) *Immunobiology of Normal and Diabetic Pregnancy*. New York: Wiley, 1990; 229

23 Dörner G, Plagemann A, Reinagel H. Familial diabetes aggregation in type 2 diabetics: gestational diabetes as apparent risk factor for increased diabetes susceptibility in the offspring. *Exp Clin Endocrinol Diabetes* 1987; **89**: 84

24 Dörner G, Steindel E, Thoelke H, Sehliak V. Evidence for decreasing prevalence of diabetes mellitus in childhood apparently produced by prevention of hyperinsulinism in the foetus and newborn. *Exp Clin Endocrinol Diabetes* 1984; **84**: 134

25 Van Assche FA. Birthweight as risk factor for breast cancer. *Lancet* 1997; **349**: 502

26 Aerts L, Holemans K, Van Assche FA. Impaired insulin response and action in offspring of severely diabetes rats. In: Shafrir E. (ed) *Frontiers in Diabetes Research. Lessons from Animal Diabetes III*. UK:Smith-Gordon,1990; 561–6

27 Kervran A, Guillaume M, Jost A. The endocrine pancreas of the fetus from diabetic pregnant rat. *Diabetologia* 1978; **15**: 387–93

28 Ktorza A, Gauguier D, Bihoreau MT, Berthault MF, Picon L. Adult offspring from mildly hyperglycemic rats show impairment of glucose regulation and insulin secretion which is transmissible to the next generation. In: Shafrir E. (ed) *Frontiers in Diabetes Research. Lessons from Animal Diabetes III*. 1990; 555–60

29 Aerts L, Vercruysse L, Van Assche FA. The endocrine pancreas in virgin and pregnant offspring of diabetic pregnant rats. *Diabetes Res Clin Pract* 1997; **38**: 9–19

30 Oh W, Gelardi NL, Cha CJ. Maternal hyperglycemia in pregnant rats: its effect on growth and carbohydrate metabolism in the offspring. *Metabolism* 1988; **37**: 1146–51

31 Susa JB, Boylan JM, Sehgal PK, Schwartz R. Impaired insulin secretion after intravenous glucose in neonatal rhesus monkeys that had been chronically hyperinsulinemic *in utero*. *Proc Soc Exp Biol Med* 1992; **199**: 327–31.

32 Plagemann A, Heidrich I, Rohde W, Gotz F, Dörner G. Hyperinsulinism during differentiation of the hypothalamus is a diabetogenic and obesity risk factor in rats. *Neuroendocrinol Lett* 1992; **5**: 373–8

33 Philipps AF, Rosenkrantz TS, Grunnet ML, Connolly ME, Porte PJ, Raye JR. Effects of fetal insulin secretory deficiency on metabolism in fetal lamb. *Diabetes* 1986; **35**: 964–72

34 Canavan JP, Goldspink DF. Maternal diabetes in rats II. Effects on fetal growth and protein turnover. *Diabetes* 1988; **37**: 1671–7

35 Aerts L, Van Bree R, Feytons V, Rombauts W, Van Assche FA. Plasma amino acids in diabetic pregnant rats and in their fetal and adult offspring. *Biol Neonate* 1989; **56**: 31–9

36 Holemans K, Aerts L, van Assche FA. Evidence for an insulin resistance in the adult offspring of streptozotocin-diabetic pregnant rats. *Diabetologia* 1991; **34**: 81–5

37 Holemans K, Van Bree R, Verhaeghe J, Aerts L, Van Assche FA. *In vivo* glucose utilization by individual tissues in virgin and pregnant offspring of severely diabetic rats. *Diabetes* 1993; **42**: 530–56

38 Ryan EA, Liu D, Bell RC, Finegood DT, Crawford J. Long term consequences in offspring of diabetes in pregnancy: studies with syngeneic islet-transplanted streptozotocin-diabetic rats. *Endocrinology* 1995; **136**: 5587–92

39 Holemans K, Aerts L, Van Assche FA. Islet transplantation in diabetic rats in mid-pregnancy does not normalize long-term effects on insulin sensitivity in adult offspring of severely diabetic pregnant rats. *J Soc Gynecol Invest* 2000; **7**: 94A (abstract 181)

40 Shoemaker JK, Bonen A. Vascular actions of insulin in health and disease. *Can J Appl Physiol* 1995; **20**: 127–54

41 Laakso M, Edelman SV, Brechtel G, Baron AD. Decreased effects of insulin to stimulate skeletal muscle blood flow in obese man: a novel mechanism for insulin resistance. *J Clin Invest* 1990; **85**: 1844–53

42 Holemans K, Gerber RT, Meurrens K, De Clerck F, Poston L, Van Assche FA. Streptozotocin diabetes in the pregnant rat induces cardiovascular dysfunction in adult offspring. *Diabetologia* 1999; **42**: 81–9

43 Johnstone MT, Creager SJ, Scales KM, Cusco JA, Lee, BK, Creager MA. Impaired endothelium-dependent vasodilation in patients with insulin-dependent diabetes mellitus. *Circulation* 1993; **88**: 2510–6

44 Taylor PD, McCarthy AL, Thomas CR, Poston L. Endothelium-dependent relaxation and noradrenaline sensitivity in mesenteric arteries of streptozotocin-induced diabetic rats. *Br J Pharmacol* 1992; **107**: 393–9

45 Goode GK, Heagerty AM. *In vitro* responses of human peripheral small arteries in hypercholesterolemia and effects of therapy. *Circulation* 1995; **91**: 2898–903

46 Girerd XJ, Hirsch AT, Cooke JP, Dzau VJ, Creager MA. L-arginine augments endothelium-dependent vasodilation in cholesterol-fed rabbits. *Circ Res* 1990; **67**: 1301–8

47 Holemans K, Aerts L, Van Assche FA. Absence of pregnancy-induced alterations in tissue insulin sensitivity in the offspring of diabetic rats. *J Endocrinol* 1991; **131**: 387–93

48 Holemans K, Gerber RT, O'Brian-Coker I, Mallet A, Van Assche FA, Poston L. Raised saturated fat intake worsens vascular function in virgin and pregnant offspring of streptozotocin-diabetic rats. *Br J Nutr* 2000; **84**: 285–96

49 Hunt JV, Dean RT, Wolff SP. Hydroxyl radical production and autoxidative glycosylation: glucose autoxidation as the cause of protein damage in the experimental glycation model of diabetes mellitus and ageing. *Biochem J* 1988; **256**: 205–12

50 Aerts L, Van Assche FA. Is gestational diabetes an acquired condition ? *J Dev Physiol* 1979; **1**: 219–25

51 Barker DJP. Fetal origins of coronary heart disease. *BMJ* 1995; **311**: 171–4

52 Phillips DI, Barker DJP, Hales CN, Hirst S, Osmond C. Thinness at birth and insulin resistance in adult life. *Diabetologia* 1994; **37**: 150

53 Reusens-Billen B, Remacle C, Hoet JJ. The development of the fetal rat intestine and its reaction to maternal diabetes II. Effect of mild and severe maternal diabetes. *Diabetes Res Clin Pract* 1989; **6**: 213

54 Stern MP, Bartley M, Duggirala R, Bradshaw B. Birth weight and the metabolic syndrome: thrifty phenotype or thrifty genotype ? *Diabetes Metab Res Rev* 2000; **16**: 88–93

Potential for the prevention of type 2 diabetes

Johan Eriksson, Jaana Lindström and Jaakko Tuomilehto

Diabetes and Genetic Epidemiology Unit, Department of Epidemiology and Health Promotion, National Public Health Institute, Helsinki, Finland

Need for prevention and prevention strategies

Type 2 diabetes is one of the most rapidly increasing chronic diseases in the world. The need for its primary prevention has been increasingly emphasised, although only during the past 10–15 years[1–6]. The main justifications of prevention of type 2 diabetes are the possible prevention or postponement of complications related to type 2 diabetes in order to reduce both human suffering and the socio-economic burden on the community. It has been repeatedly shown that both symptomatic and asymptomatic diabetic patients have an increased prevalence of both macrovascular and microvascular complications by the time the disease is first diagnosed[7–9]. A Swedish study showed that 77% of all costs for the care of type 2 diabetes were due to its complications, mostly cardio-vascular[10]. Also, in people with impaired glucose tolerance (IGT), both mortality and the risk of cardiovascular disease are markedly increased[11,12]. It has been estimated that at the time of diagnosis of clinical type 2 diabetes only 50–60% of the pancreatic β-cell capacity is left, due to the fact that the disease process has already existed for more than 10 years[13]. Therefore, the optimal (and probably the only effective) strategy to reduce the increased burden of type 2 diabetes is primary prevention, *i.e.* to tackle the worsening of glucose intolerance before harmful effects of hyperglycaemia become permanent.

The increased knowledge about the aetiology, pathogenesis and natural history of type 2 diabetes has lead to primary prevention becoming a reality. Although an unequivocally accepted consensus regarding the early pathogenesis is still lacking, preventive measures can be based upon the best current available knowledge. The rapidly increasing number of patients with type 2 diabetes, the severity of the disease, its multiple and severe complications and the increasing socio-economic costs emphasise the importance of immediate preventive actions. The current situation for type 2 diabetes can be compared with the epidemic of coronary heart disease during the 1960s and 1970s in many industrialised countries[14–16]. Primary preventive measures targeted at the known modifiable risk

Correspondence to:
Dr Jaana Lindström,
Diabetes and Genetic
Epidemiology Unit,
Department of
Epidemiology and Health
Promotion, National
Public Health Institute,
Mannerheimintie 166,
FIN-00300 Helsinki,
Finland

factors of coronary heart disease have shown to be successful. Both the incidence and mortality of coronary heart diseases and stroke have halved in about 20 years, though the extent to which this reflects the success of preventive policies is not known[17].

Primary prevention of type 2 diabetes can be defined as all measures designed to reduce the incidence of the disease on the population level, by reducing the risk of its onset. This may be achieved by modifying the underlying risk factors for type 2 diabetes. Secondary prevention of type 2 diabetes can be defined as all measures designed to reduce morbidity and mortality among diagnosed type 2 diabetic patients.

Prevention strategies

Since type 2 diabetes is a heterogeneous and multifactorial disorder, preventive measures must be based upon modification of several risk factors simultaneously. Otherwise, the potential for prevention remains incomplete and insufficient. The existing evidence, however, suggests that even a single intervention, *e.g.* increased physical activity in sedentary people or weight loss in the obese, can lead to a marked reduction in the risk of type 2 diabetes[18,19] There are two components to the design of a prevention strategy: (i) a population-based strategy, for altering the life-style and those environmental determinants which are the underlying causes of type 2 diabetes in the entire population; and (ii) a high-risk strategy for screening individuals at high risk for type 2 diabetes and bringing preventive measures to this group on an individual basis.

The basic underlying principle of the population approach is to shift the average blood glucose concentration of the whole population in the direction of lower values, or to prevent the increase in blood glucose with age. The population strategy and the high-risk strategy are, however, complementary and one of them may not be effective without the other being applied simultaneously. The primary emphasis on the population approach may be more appropriate in societies with a particularly high susceptibility to type 2 diabetes, while the emphasis on the high-risk strategy may be more appropriate in communities with a moderate risk. Since the frequency of the disease is increasing steeply in most populations in the world, the population approach needs to be considered as a priority.

According to present knowledge, the known high risk individuals are: (i) those with a family history of type 2 diabetes; (ii) women who had gestational diabetes; (iii) people whose blood glucose has been previously found to be moderately increased; and (iv) hypertensive subjects. In addition, obese and physically inactive people have an increased risk for type 2 diabetes. Altogether, these high-risk individuals are so numerous in modern societies that they would in fact comprise a large proportion of the adult population world-wide. As knowledge of the genetic predisposition for type 2 diabetes increases, communities with a high genetic predisposition should be targeted.

Natural history of type 2 diabetes – the basis for prevention

Primary prevention of type 2 diabetes depends on our current know-ledge of the natural history of the disease. It is known that type 2 diabetes has a strong genetic predisposition[4]. In addition, recent findings point towards the importance of events during fetal life and infancy. It has been hypothesised that fetal experience, such as malnutrition, can lead to programming of the metabolic profile that will contribute to the development of chronic diseases in adult life, including type 2 diabetes[20]. This early programming mimics to a great extent 'genetic' transmission of diseases. When predisposed individuals become more insulin resistant, for example due to obesity or physical inactivity in their adult life, they usually develop some degree of glucose intolerance. When the pancreatic β-cell capacity is no longer sufficient to compensate for the increasing insulin production needed to overcome insulin resistance, hyperglycaemia worsens and overt diabetes develops. It is important to understand that progression through these stages is not inevitable – it is probable that this progression can be halted and actually was halted in years past when populations were less obese and more physically active. Potentially, intervention at any stage of the natural history of diabetes may prevent the progression to a later stage of glucose intolerance.

When does the clock start ticking for type 2 diabetes?

The clock starts ticking for diabetes long before any abnormalities can be detected. A number of stages relating to the course and development of type 2 diabetes may be defined. The data from the UK prospective diabetes study showed that, at the time of the diagnosis of type 2 diabetes, 50% of the overall β-cell function had already been lost[13]. From the further linear deterioration of the β-cell capacity in these diabetic patients, it was estimated that the β-cell capacity had begun to decline ~12 years prior to the clinical diagnosis of diabetes. The first stage in this process is genetic susceptibility. Another very early component that may contribute to the predisposition is the disproportionate body size at birth, that is thinness or macrosomia at birth. These can be readily identified and may be considered as the first identifiable risk indicator, especially in families with a history of diabetes. In the general population, however, general cut-off points for thinness or fatness vary within populations and have yet to be defined.

It is well established that an abnormal intra-uterine environment leads to structural and functional adaptations in the fetus which have long-lasting consequences for its metabolism in later life. A thesis of this book is that a thrifty phenotype develops in which inadequate fetal nutrition programmes impaired development of glucose and insulin metabolism in adulthood[21]. Disproportionate size at birth is a fairly recently discovered risk factor in the list of risk factors for type 2 diabetes. The proposed biological mechanisms involve both pancreatic β-cell dysfunction and insulin resistance; therefore, the associations are highly plausible given the multiple observational studies and animal experiments that support them.

British studies originally showed that babies born with the lightest birth weight, *i.e.* < 2.5 kg, were almost 7 times more likely to have some degree of impairment in their glucose tolerance compared with those born heavier[22]. Similar findings have now been made globally in a variety of populations and ethnic groups[23-25]. In keeping with the thrifty phenotype hypothesis are also findings from twin studies; the twin with type 2 diabetes has lower birth weight[26]. Monozygotic twins share the same genetic make-up, suggesting that the mechanism of the link between low birth weight and subsequent type 2 diabetes is environmental. This should not lead to the conclusion that the there is no role for genetics in the development of type 2 diabetes, but it certainly shows that the link between low birth weight and type 2 diabetes can occur independently of a genetic influence. The thrifty phenotype hypothesis has been challenged by McCance and co-workers who described a U-shaped relationship between birth weight and type 2 diabetes among Pima Indians[27]. The risk of type 2 diabetes in infants weighing <2.5 kg at birth was 3.8 times that of infants weighing 2.5–4.5 kg whereas those with birth weights >4.5 kg had a 1.8-fold increased relative risk. The increased risk associated with higher birth weight could in fact be due to the high prevalence of type 2 diabetes among the Pima Indians and consequently high prevalence of gestational diabetes and macrosomia in the offspring.

The importance of exposures before birth on the life-time occurrence of chronic diseases has recently been shown in many populations and for many diseases[20]. In the past, when infectious diseases were more common, it was evident that childhood health affected health in adult life. Now the current observations also stress the importance of fetal life as a crucial period for the natural history of type 2 diabetes.

Growth in childhood and adolescence

The thrifty phenotype hypothesis suggests that the fetal nutritional environment has a programming effect on various physiological functions including glucose and lipid metabolism and blood pressure[20]. It is the mismatch between a relatively poor intra-uterine environment and a nutritionally rich environment in later life that increases the risk of diabetes and other diseases. Adaptation to undernutrition *in utero* may limit the extent of dietary change to which a generation can be exposed without adverse effects. Individuals exposed to undernutrition *in utero* are more susceptible to type 2 diabetes if they catch-up in weight and body mass index (BMI) during childhood as shown by a recent study in Finland[25]. Since children born small and thin have proportionally less muscle mass, catch-up growth would mean disproportionate increase in weight and fat mass in relation to muscle and height during early childhood. Therefore, prevention of obesity during childhood is important among children born small and thin.

Recently, an alarming rise in the incidence of type 2 diabetes among children and adolescents in the US has been observed, though this is not limited to North America[28,29]. As the young population world-wide is becoming increasingly overweight and sedentary, type 2 diabetes will probably appear more frequently in younger age groups than before. Puberty appears to play a major role in the development of diabetes in children. During puberty, there is increased resistance to the action of insulin, resulting in hyperinsulinaemia which contributes to the manifestation of both type 1 and type 2 diabetes. One underlying cause of this could be increased growth hormone secretion, and this effect is modified by obesity[20]. It is commonly understood that subjects with an early-onset type 2 diabetes probably have a stronger genetic predisposition than those diabetic patients whose onset age is older. The recent increase observed in the prevalence of type 2 diabetes in younger age groups has, however, occurred too rapidly to be the result of an increased gene frequency and altered genetic pool, emphasising the importance of environmental factors that can trigger the disease onset in genetically predisposed people.

Health habits and their 'programming' in youth

Another important aspect of fetal programming is the 'programming' of life-style. Children readily adopt the life-style of their parents. Childhood and adolescence are periods in life during which they also tend to adopt the life-styles of their peers. This is the first period when knowledge and awareness of type 2 diabetes and its risk factors should be disseminated to the population. Primarily, the preventive message should include aspects related to practical advice regarding a healthy diet and the promotion of physical activity; it should be targeted to the entire population, not only to high risk individuals. The 'peer pressure' among the youth is so strong that benefits expected from such a population approach to control environmental risk factors for type 2 diabetes are likely to be substantial.

Adult life-style

The epidemic of obesity can be viewed as the result of a normal response to an abnormal environment. In 1985, the World Health Organization named obesity the single most important risk factor for type 2 diabetes[30]. This is evident since it has been estimated[31] that up to two-thirds of type 2 diabetes could be prevented by keeping the BMI < 25 kg/m^2. The increase in obesity in adults is partly explained by a decrease in physical activity, but sedentary life-style is also an independent risk factor for type 2 diabetes[4,32]. The combination of 'Westernisation' and genetic predisposition for type 2 diabetes can result in an epidemic of type 2 diabetes even within one generation as seen in some populations such as Pima Indians and Nauruans[33]. Therefore, it would be necessary to set a target in the population as well as for individuals to maintain the level of body weight as it was around the age of 25 years and also to maintain a sufficient level of physical activity throughout adult life. By applying these simple measures, more than half of the cases of type 2 diabetes occurring before the age of 65 years could be prevented.

Elderly individuals

The occurrence of type 2 diabetes increases with increasing age, and the vast majority of diabetic subjects are elderly. There are physiological reasons for this and they are largely related to life-style. Muscle mass usually decreases with advanced age. To what extent this can be considered as a part of a normal ageing process and to what extent it is due to an increase in sedentary life-style with age is not fully settled. Also, various musculoskeletal problems increase with age and often affect exercise habits. It is probable that some exposures during the intra-uterine period and early infancy may prevent normal β-cell growth and replication leading to a permanently reduced β-cell capacity. The pancreatic β-cell mass decreases with age. This process is accelerated by peripheral insulin resistance due to influences such as obesity, physical inactivity, and diet. In people who are genetically susceptible to diabetes, this process leads to hyperglycaemia and, ultimately, to clinical diabetes. The tempo of this development and hence the age-at-onset of disease are obviously determined by the intensity of environmental exposure. This is well illustrated by the increasing number of type 2 diabetics among adolescents and young adults[34].

Identification of target groups for intervention and implementation of preventive measures

Family history

Family history is one of the most important determinants of type 2 diabetes. The currently accepted pathogenic model for type 2 diabetes is based upon the assumption that a genetic predisposition is necessary, but not a sufficient cause, for the disease. Thus, type 2 diabetes may only develop in individuals who carry diabetes susceptibility genes. Since in some populations such as Native Americans and Pacific Islanders, the life-time prevalence of type 2 diabetes is now over 50%, it can be assumed that more than half of people in these populations are genetically predisposed to diabetes[3]. It has been suggested that 'thrifty genotypes' have accumulated in such isolated populations[35]. Similarly, epidemiological studies from Europid populations show that 20–30% of people aged 70 years or above have type 2 diabetes[36]. Thus, at least this proportion of Europid populations carry susceptibility genes. Assuming a Mendelian inheritance, at least half of their siblings and offspring should also have these genes.

Twin studies have suggested that the majority of monozygotic twin pairs will become concordant for type 2 diabetes after one twin develops the disease. The concordance estimates vary between 60–100%[37]. Our own twin study has revealed that approximately half of the liability to type 2 diabetes is related to genetic effects and a half to environmental exposure[38].

Previously, family history has not been found to be a sensitive marker for the disease for three reasons: (i) almost half of the first degree relatives of type 2 diabetic patients have not inherited the susceptibility genes; (ii) the majority of those genetically predisposed do not develop diabetes either because of low exposure to environmental risk factors or through premature mortality from other causes; and (iii) diabetic subjects in the past were often not properly diagnosed[39]. While the first reason is still relevant, the latter two have drastically changed, but still remain relevant. Looking at the importance of family history from the other perspective, a positive evidence for family history of type 2 diabetes is always an indication for at least a 50% probability of diabetes risk for an individual.

Low birth weight

Type 2 diabetes has been shown to be associated with intra-uterine or early childhood malnutrition. One might, therefore, predict that the incidence of type 2 diabetes will fall as the nutritional status in a population and in pregnant women improves. Nevertheless, adequate fetal nutrition may not offset the effects of diabetes susceptibility genes. The protein metabolism of women during pregnancy is closely related to the glucose-insulin metabolism of the offspring, and the importance of essential amino acids in programming the fetus has been stressed. However, fetal growth is not only regulated by the availability of nutrients but by hormones, growth factors, and placental functions.

It would be helpful to know what proportion of type 2 diabetes is the result of early growth retardation. Birth weight, however, is a crude index of fetal growth and development, and there is a continuous relationship – rather than a threshold – between birth weight and the future risk of type 2 diabetes[20]. Furthermore, early catch-up growth and childhood obesity interact with an intra-uterine exposure making this matter complex[25]. Low birth weight can serve as a surrogate marker for intra-uterine exposure and is a risk factor for type 2 diabetes which should be considered at least in people with a positive family history. It would be interesting to examine the glucose tolerance status of individuals with optimal early growth. This might reveal a potential way to prevent type 2 diabetes. We do not yet know whether and to what extent improvements in the body compositions and diets of young women can contribute to the primary prevention of type 2 diabetes in their offspring.

Childhood obesity

Attempts to prevent type 2 diabetes in children should follow the same general paradigm as that recommended for the prevention of type 2 diabetes in adults. Although primary prevention efforts may be directed at high-risk individuals, the main strategy must be based up on applying prevention strategies at the population level.

Prevention of type 2 diabetes in high-risk children is predicated on the ability to identify those at increased risk and provide them with adequate service. The population approach should promote the avoidance of obesity and adequate levels of physical activity as desired norms for the entire community. These objectives may not be easy to achieve in the real world, but they are not unreasonable.

In addition to overall health promotion in the community at large, there is a need for health professionals to become involved in developing and implementing school- and community-based programmes to promote improved dietary and physical activity behaviours for all children as well as their families. School programmes should promote healthy food choices and increased physical activity.

Gestational diabetes

Gestational diabetes, or hyperglycaemia occurring temporarily during pregnancy, is associated with an increased risk of the later development of type 2 diabetes. The 15-year cumulative incidence is 35–40% or 3–5% per year[40]. Gestational diabetes is not only associated with an increased risk of diabetes in the mother, but with an increased risk of diabetes in the offspring (see Van Assche *et al*, this issue). Proper weight management and the promotion of physical activity in these women is essential in order to prevent the development of overt diabetes later in life. Women with previous gestational diabetes are one of the target groups whose glucose tolerance should be systematically monitored.

Hypertension

It is known that people with hypertension have more diabetes than normotensive subjects[41,42], and the risk of cardiovascular disease in hypertensive diabetic patients is particularly high[43]. Therefore, it is important to determine the glucose tolerance status in hypertensive patients at regular intervals. While the control of blood pressure among patients treated for hypertension is often inadequate[44], several studies have demonstrated that hypertensive diabetic patients seem to benefit especially from lowering of their blood pressure[45,46].

Adult obesity

A close association between obesity and type 2 diabetes has been observed in both cross-sectional and prospective studies[47–52]. Even modest degrees of overweight increase the risk of type 2 diabetes. Obesity and physical inactivity are the most important potentially modifiable risk factors for type 2 diabetes. Based upon epidemiological data, it has been estimated that the risk of type 2 diabetes could be reduced by 50–75% by control of obesity and by 30–50% by increasing physical activity[31]. Preventive measures during adulthood should primarily focus on weight management and increase in physical activity.

Transiently or slightly elevated blood glucose

In general, there are a number of stages relating to the course and development of type 2 diabetes. The earliest stage of detectable abnormality in glucose homeostasis is impaired glucose tolerance (IGT), *i.e.* elevated postprandial blood glucose concentrations[53]. According to different studies, 2–5% of people with IGT will develop frank diabetes. Though a large proportion of people with IGT will have normal glucose tolerance on a repeat test[54], it has been shown that many of them will later on have IGT again and will ultimately develop diabetes[55]; however, progression is not inevitable. The probability in worsening from IGT to diabetes is related to life-style factors such as obesity and physical inactivity. From the prevention point of view IGT is a critical stage in the development of diabetes, because it is readily detectable and treatment may prevent or delay its progression.

Past experience from primary prevention of diabetes mellitus

Even though primary prevention of diabetes was first proposed 80 years ago[56] and more recently stressed by the WHO[57], few studies have attempted to assess the value of measures aimed at controlling obesity and increasing physical activity in people with a high risk of the disease. Some intervention studies have used drugs but these studies will not be considered here since such intervention cannot be considered as primary prevention. An intervention programme based solely on life-style intervention is a natural way of preventing type 2 diabetes since the increased prevalence and incidence of the disease is mainly due to responses to a sedentary life-style and excessive food intake.

Unfortunately the published life-style intervention studies have not been properly designed or powered to give a definite answer to the question of whether or to what extent the primary prevention of type 2 diabetes is possible. However some have provided suggestive evidence that life-style changes are effective in halting the progression from IGT to type 2 diabetes. We will briefly summarise the main findings from these studies.

The feasibility of diet and exercise intervention in 217 men with IGT was assessed in the Malmö feasibility study[18]. The effect of exercise and diet was compared to a reference group with no intervention. The reference group consisted of men who themselves decided not to join the intervention programme. Thus, the groups were not assigned at random. By the end of the 5-year study period, 11% of the intervention group and 21% of the reference group had developed diabetes. Thus the incidence in the intervention group was a half of that in the reference group (RR, 0.5; 95% CI, 0.3–1.0). This study is important in demonstrating the feasibility of carrying out a diet-exercise programme for 5-years among volunteers.

More recently, data on the preventive effect of a diet and exercise intervention have been reported in a cluster-randomised clinical trial on

577 subjects with IGT in Da-Qing, China[19]. The cumulative 6-year incidence of type 2 diabetes was notably lower in the three (diet alone, exercise alone, diet-exercise combined) intervention groups, being 41–46% compared with 68% in the control group. This study did not apply an individual allocation of study subjects to the intervention and control groups; instead the participating clinics were allocated. Thus, the study unit was a clinic not a person and, therefore, the results based on individual data must be interpreted with caution. Furthermore, the study subjects were relatively lean, with a mean BMI of 25.8 kg/m^2, making inferences to European obese IGT subjects difficult. Also, the rate of progression from IGT to diabetes was unusually high, more than 10% per year in the control group, which exceeds that usually reported in observational studies[58].

Promising results on the treatment of obesity come from the Swedish SOS Intervention Study[59]. The 2-year incidence of diabetes was 30 times lower in surgically treated, grossly obese subjects compared to control subjects receiving regular care. The corresponding weight losses were 28 ± 15 kg *versus* 0.5 ± 8.9 kg ($P < 0.0001$), respectively. These results certainly suggest that severe obesity can and should be treated, and that the reduction of obesity results in a marked reduction in the incidence of hypertension, diabetes and some lipid disturbances.

There are some 'natural' experiments available in which ethnic groups have experienced rapid Westernization and with it rapid increase in the rates of obesity and type 2 diabetes. Therefore, it is logical to assume that by reversing these life-style changes it would be possible to prevent the development of the disease. Such a potential for reversibility has in fact been shown by elegant life-style intervention studies in Australian Aboriginals by O'Dea and co-workers[60]. In these experiments, when hyperglycaemic people returned to nature and lived a traditional hunter–gatherer way of life, hyperglycaemia was reversed.

Major recent life-style intervention studies

The Finnish Diabetes Prevention Study (DPS)

This was carried out between 1992–2000 in 5 clinics in different parts of Finland, aimed at preventing type 2 diabetes with life-style modification alone[61–63]. A total of 522 individuals at high risk of developing diabetes were recruited into the study, mainly by opportunistic screening for impaired glucose tolerance (IGT) in middle-aged (age, 40–64 years), overweight (BMI >25 kg/m^2) subjects. The presence of IGT was confirmed in two successive 75 g oral glucose tolerance tests; the mean of the two values had to be within the IGT range. From previous studies, it was estimated that the cumulative diabetes incidence in such a high-risk group would be 35% in 6 years. The study subjects were randomly allocated either into the control group or the intensive intervention group. The subjects in the intervention group had frequent consultation visits with a nutritionist and received individual advice to reduce weight and dietary intake of total and saturated fat, and to increase fibre intake. They were advised to increase everyday activity and were offered supervised, circuit-type exercise sessions aiming to increase muscle mass in addition to aerobic exercise. The control group subjects were also given general advice about healthy life-style at their annual visits to the study clinic. An oral glucose tolerance test was done annually and, in the case of diabetic values, a confirmatory OGTT was performed.

During the first year of the study, body weight decreased on average 4.2 kg in the intervention group and 0.8 kg in the control group subjects ($P = 0.0001$). Most of the weight reduction was maintained during the second year. Also, indicators of central adiposity and fasting glucose and insulin, 2-h post-challenge glucose and insulin, and HbA1c reduced significantly, more in the intervention group than in the control group at both 1-year and 2-year follow-up examinations. At the 1-year and 2-year examinations, intervention group subjects reported significantly more beneficial changes in their dietary and exercise habits, based on dietary and exercise diaries.

A total of 86 incident cases of diabetes were diagnosed among the 522 subjects after a median follow-up duration of 3 years. Of these, 27 occurred in the intervention group and 59 in the control group. The cumulative incidence in the intervention group was 58% lower than in the control group (Fig. 1).

The difference between the groups became statistically significant after 2 years: 6% in the intervention group and 14% in the control group. At 4 years, the cumulative incidences were 11% and 23%, respectively. The absolute risk of diabetes was 32/1000 person-years in the intervention group and 78/1000 person-years in the control group. In men, the incidence of diabetes was reduced by 63% in the intervention group compared with the control group and in women by 54%.

According to these results, 22 people with IGT need to be treated for 1 year or 5 people for 5 years with a life-style intervention to prevent one case of diabetes. The public health implications of these results are wide. The primary prevention of type 2 diabetes is possible by a non-pharmacological intervention that can be implemented in the primary health care setting. It is necessary that such an intervention becomes part of routine preventive care in order to reduce the burden of type 2 diabetes that is reaching epidemic proportions in many countries. At the same time, it is also necessary to develop national programmes for the

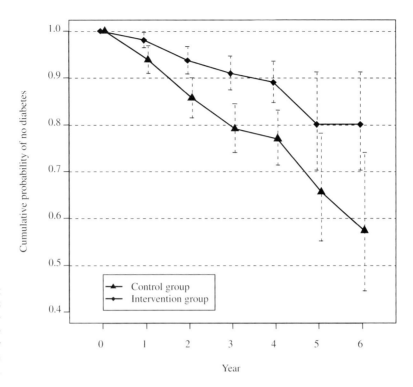

Fig. 1 Development of diabetes in subjects with IGT at baseline during the life-style intervention trial by the randomisation group[63].

primary prevention of type 2 diabetes that include not only the high risk strategy but also the population strategy.

The Diabetes Prevention Program (DPP)

This was a randomised clinical trial comparing the efficacy and safety of three interventions – an intensive life-style intervention, or standard life-style recommendations combined with either metformin or placebo[64]. The study focused on high-risk individuals with elevated fasting plasma glucose and impaired glucose tolerance ($n = 3234$). The original closing date of the study was planned to be 2002. However, the study was terminated prematurely by the external data monitoring board because the data had clearly answered the main research questions[65]. Intensive life-style intervention, with 58% reduction in type 2 diabetes risk compared to the placebo group, was superior to the metformin group with 31% reduction in diabetes risk, and the DPP study confirmed the results obtained in the Finnish DPS study. The life-style intervention was done by special educators, not regular health personnel, and was intense. Thus, the translation of such intervention to a routine primary health care may not be easy.

The future

Primary prevention of type 2 diabetes needs to receive more serious attention than in the past. Even though the WHO Study Group in 1994 gave a strong recommendation that national diabetes prevention programmes should be set up, none has been initiated thus far. A plethora of observational data demonstrates that life-style factors including physical inactivity and obesity are increasing throughout the world and that these trends have been accompanied with the steep increase in type 2 diabetes. These unfavourable life-style patterns are not only an issue among adults but also among children and adolescents. As a consequence, the age-at-onset of type 2 diabetes has become younger, not only in special small ethnic groups like Pima Indians but in many societies in both industrialised and non-industrialised countries. The effect of these life-style patterns is particularly deleterious in those born small and thin and who had accelerated weight gain during childhood and adolescence.

Data from intervention studies in various settings provide unequivocal evidence that the risk of type 2 diabetes in high-risk individuals can be reversed. While it is useful to accumulate more information from interventions in other populations and cultural environments, the evidence for initiating intensive actions to prevent type 2 diabetes is clearly sufficient. The identification of high-risk subjects for type 2 diabetes is relatively easy; biochemical or other costly tests are not required, and most of the high-risk subjects are already regular customers of primary health care services. What is needed is the systematic approach to target life-style intervention to these individuals. This is not an easy task, but we know for instance from cardiovascular prevention programmes that such interventions are possible and efficient[66].

Interventions in high-risk subjects alone will not be sufficient for the successful prevention of type 2 diabetes; it is necessary to initiate actions based on the population approach. The co-ordinated combination of the high-risk approach together with systematic population approaches are likely to be the most efficient strategy. Action is overdue and is only now being begun in some countries. The national consensus conference on diabetes control in Finland in 2000 listed the primary prevention of type 2 diabetes as the primary issue among all activities in diabetes care. A programme is currently being developed. Other countries are likely to develop similar activities in the near future. In such programmes, it is necessary to realise that the primary prevention of type 2 diabetes requires a long-term plan and must include a range of activities targeted at different age groups from fetal life to old age.

References

1   Tuomilehto J, Wolf E. Primary prevention of diabetes mellitus. *Diabetes Care* 1987; **10**: 238–48
2   King H, Dowd JE. Primary prevention of type 2 (non-insulin-dependent) diabetes mellitus. *Diabetologia* 1990; **33**: 3–8

3   Tuomilehto J, Tuomilehto-Wolf E, Zimmet P, Alberti K, Knowler W. Primary prevention of diabetes mellitus. In: Alberti K, Zimmet P, DeFronzo R, Keen H. (eds) *International Textbook of Diabetes Mellitus*, 2nd edn. Chichester: Wiley, 1997; 1799–827

4   Hamman RF. Genetic and environmental determinants of non-insulin-dependent diabetes mellitus (NIDDM). *Diabetes Metab Rev* 1992; **8**: 287–338

5   Zimmet PZ. Primary prevention of diabetes mellitus. *Diabetes Care* 1988; **11**: 258–62

6   Stern MP. Primary prevention of type II diabetes mellitus. *Diabetes Care* 1991; **14**: 399–410

7   Haffner S, Mykkänen L, Festa A, Burke J, Stern M. Insulin-resistant prediabetic subjects have more atherogenic risk factors than insulin-sensitive prediabetic subjects: implications for preventing coronary heart disease during prediabetic state. *Circulation* 2000; **101**: 975–80

8   Harris M, Klein R, Welborn T, Knuiman M. Onset of NIDDM occurs at least 4–7 years before clinical diagnosis. *Diabetes Care* 1992; **15**: 815–9

9   Uusitupa M, Siitonen O, Aro A, Pyörälä K. Prevalence of coronary heart disease, left ventricular failure and hypertension in middle-aged, newly diagnosed type 2 (non-insulin-dependent) diabetic subjects. *Diabetologia* 1985; **28**: 22–7

10   Henriksson F, Agardh C, Berne C *et al*. Direct medical costs for patients with type 2 diabetes in Sweden. *J Intern Med* 2000; **248**: 387–96

11   The DECODE Study Group. Glucose tolerance and mortality: comparison of WHO and American Diabetes Association diagnostic criteria. *Lancet* 1999; **354**: 617–21

12   Tominaga M, Eguchi H, Manaka H, Igarashi K, Kato T, Sekikawa A. Impaired glucose tolerance is a risk factor for cardiovascular disease, but not impaired fasting glucose. *Diabetes Care* 1999; **22**: 920–4

13   UKPDS Group. UK prospective diabetes study 16: overview of six years' therapy of type 2 diabetes – a progressive disease. *Diabetes* 1995; **44**: 1249–58

14   Keys A. *Coronary Heart Disease in Seven Countries*. New York: American Heart Association, 1970

15   Uemura K, Pisa Z. Trends in cardiovascular disease mortality in industrialized countries since 1950. *World Health Stat Q* 1988; **41**: 155–78

16   Sarti C, Rastenyte D, Cepaitis Z, Tuomilehto J. International trends in mortality from stroke 1968 to 1994. *Stroke* 2000; **31**: 1588–601

17   Kuulasmaa K, Tunstall-Pedoe H, Dobson A *et al*. Estimation of contribution of changes in classic risk factors to trends in coronary-event rates across the WHO MONICA Project populations. *Lancet* 2000; **355**: 675–87

18   Eriksson KF, Lindgarde F. Prevention of type 2 (non-insulin-dependent) diabetes mellitus by diet and physical exercise. The 6-year Malmö feasibility study. *Diabetologia* 1991; **34**: 891–8

19   Pan XR, Li GW, Hu YH *et al*. Effects of diet and exercise in preventing NIDDM in people with impaired glucose tolerance. The Da Qing IGT and Diabetes Study. *Diabetes Care* 1997; **20**: 537–44

20   Barker D. *Mothers, Babies, and Health in Later Life*, 2nd edn. Edinburgh: Churchill Livingstone, 1998

21   Hales C, Barker D. Type 2 (non-insulin-dependent) diabetes mellitus: the thrifty phenotype hypothesis. *Diabetologia* 1992; **35**: 595–601

22   Hales C, Barker D, Clark P *et al*. Fetal and infant growth and impaired glucose tolerance at age 64. *BMJ* 1991; **303**: 1019–22

23   Lithell H, McKeigue P, Berglund L, Mohsen R, Lithell U, Leon D. Relation of size at birth to non-insulin dependent diabetes and insulin concentrations in men aged 50–60 years. *BMJ* 1996; **312**: 406–10

24   Rich-Edwards J, Colditz G, Stampfer M *et al*. Birthweight and the risk for type 2 diabetes mellitus in adult women. *Ann Intern Med* 1999; **130**: 278–84

25   Forsén T, Eriksson J, Tuomilehto J, Reunanen A, Osmond C, Barker D. The fetal and childhood growth of persons who develop type 2 diabetes. *Ann Intern Med* 2000; **133**: 176–82

26   Poulsen P, Vaag A, Kyvik K, Moller Jensen D, Beck-Nielsen H. Low birth weight is associated with NIDDM in discordant monozygotic and dizygotic twin pairs. *Diabetologia* 1997; **40**: 439–46

27   McCance D, Pettitt D, Hanson R, Jacobsson L, Knowler W, Bennett P. Birth weight and non-insulin dependent diabetes: thrifty genotype, thrifty phenotype, or surviving small baby

genotype? *BMJ* 1994; **308**: 942–5

28   American Diabetes Association. Type 2 diabetes in children and adolescents. *Diabetes Care* 2000; **23**: 381–9

29   Reilly J, Dorosty A. Epidemic of obesity in UK children. *Lancet* 1999; **354**: 1874–5

30   WHO Study Group. *Diabetes Mellitus – Technical Report Series No 727*. Geneva; WHO, 1985

31   Manson JE, Nathan DM, Krolewski AS, Stampfer MJ, Willett WC, Hennekens CH. A prospective study of exercise and incidence of diabetes among US male physicians. *JAMA* 1992; **268**: 63–7

32   Manson JE, Rimm EB, Stampfer MJ *et al*. Physical activity and incidence of non-insulin-dependent diabetes mellitus in women. *Lancet* 1991; **338**: 774–8

33   De Courten M, Bennet P, Tuomilehto J, Zimmet P. Epidemiology in NIDDM in non-Europids. In: Alberti K, Zimmet P, DeFronzo R, Keen H. (eds) *International Textbook of Diabetes Mellitus*, 2nd edn. London: Wiley, 1997; 143–70

34   Fagot-Campagna A, Pettitt D, Engelgau M *et al*. Type 2 diabetes among North American children and adolescents: an epidemiologic review and a public health perspective. *J Pediatr* 2000; **136**: 664–72

35   Neel JV. Diabetes mellitus: a 'thrifty' genotype rendered detrimental by progress? *Am J Hum Genet* 1962; **14**: 353–62

36   Valle T, Tuomilehto J, Eriksson J. Epidemiology of type 2 diabetes in Europids. In: Alberti K, Zimmet P, DeFronzo R, Keen H. (eds) *International Textbook of Diabetes Mellitus*, 2nd edn. London: Wiley, 1997; 125–42

37   Lo S, Tun R, Hawa M, Leslie R. Studies of diabetic twins. *Diabetes Metab Rev* 1991; **7**: 223–38

38   Kaprio J, Tuomilehto J, Koskenvuo M *et al*. Concordance for type 1 (insulin-dependent) and type 2 (non-insulin-dependent) diabetes mellitus in a population-based cohort of twins in Finland. *Diabetologia* 1992; **35**: 1060–7

39   Harris M. Undiagnosed NIDDM; clinical and public health issues. *Diabetes Care* 1993; **16**: 642–52

40   Dornhorst A, Rossi M. Risk and prevention of type 2 diabetes in women with gestational diabetes. *Diabetes Care* 1998; **21 (Suppl 2)**: B43–9

41   Kannel W, Wilson P, Zhang T. The epidemiology of impaired glucose tolerance and hypertension. *Am Heart J* 1991; **121**: 1268–73

42   Reaven G, Lithell H, Landsberg L. Hypertension and associated metabolic abnormalities: role of insulin resistance and the sympathoadrenal system. *N Engl J Med* 1996; **334**: 374–81

43   Grossman E, Messerli F. Diabetic and hypertensive heart disease. *Ann Intern Med* 1996; **125**: 304–10

44   Marques-Vidal P, Tuomilehto J. Hypertension awareness, treatment and control in the community: Is the 'rule of halves' still valid. *J Hum Hypertens* 1997; **11**: 213–20

45   Tuomilehto J, Rastenyte D, Birkenhänger W *et al*. Effects of calcium-channel blockade in older patients with diabetes and systolic hypertension. *N Engl J Med* 1999; **340**: 677–84

46   UK Prospective Diabetes Study Group. Tight blood pressure control and risk of macrovascular and microvascular complications in type 2 diabetes: UKPDS 38. *BMJ* 1998; **317**: 703–13

47   West K. *Epidemiology of Diabetes and its Vascular Lesions*. New York: Elsevier, 1978

48   Medalie JH, Papier CM, Herman JB *et al*. Diabetes mellitus among 10,000 adult men: I. Five-year incidence and associated variables. *Isr J Med Sci* 1974; **10**: 681–97

49   Ohlson LO, Larsson B, Björntorp P *et al*. Risk factors for type 2 (non-insulin-dependent) diabetes mellitus: thirteen and one-half years of follow-up of the participants in a study of Swedish men born in 1913. *Diabetologia* 1988; **31**: 798–805

50   Chan JM, Rimm EB, Colditz GA, Stampfer MJ, Willett WC. Obesity, fat distribution, and weight gain as risk factors for clinical diabetes in men. *Diabetes Care* 1994; **17**: 961–9

51   Han T, Feskens E, Lean M, Seidell J. Association of body composition with type 2 diabetes mellitus. *Diabet Med* 1998; **15**: 129–35

52   Folsom A, Kushi L, Anderson K, Mink P, Olson J, Hong C-P. Association of general and abdominal obesity with multiple outcomes in older women. *Arch Intern Med* 2000; **160**: 2117–28

53   WHO Expert Committee. *Diabetes mellitus. Second report. WHO Technical Report No.: 727*. Geneva: WHO, 1980

54 Yudkin J, Alberti K, McLarty D, Swai A. Impaired glucose tolerance. Is it a risk factor for diabetes or a diagnostic ragbag? *BMJ* 1990; **301**: 397–401

55 Saad M, Knowler W, Pettitt D, Nelson R, Bennett P. Transient impaired glucose tolerance in Pima Indians? *BMJ* 1988; **297**: 1438–41

56 Joslin E. The prevention of diabetes mellitus. *JAMA* 1921; **76**: 79–84

57 WHO Study Group. *Primary prevention of diabetes mellitus – Technical Report Series No 844*. Geneva; WHO, 1994

58 Knowler W, Narayan K, Hanson R *et al*. Perspectives in diabetes. Preventing non-insulin-dependent diabetes. *Diabetes* 1995; **44**: 483–8

59 Sjöström CD, Lissner L, Wedel H, Sjöström L. Reduction in incidence of diabetes, hypertension and lipid disturbances after intentional weight loss induced by bariatric surgery: the SOS Intervention Study. *Obes Res* 1999; **7**: 477–84

60 O'Dea K. Marked improvement in carbohydrate and lipid metabolism in diabetic Australian Aborigines after temporary reversion to traditional lifestyle. *Diabetes* 1980; **33**: 596–603

61 Eriksson J, Lindström J, Valle T *et al*. Prevention of type II diabetes in subjects with impaired glucose tolerance: the Diabetes Prevention Study (DPS) in Finland – study design and 1-year interim report on the feasibility of the lifestyle intervention programme. *Diabetologia* 1999; **42**: 793–801

62 Uusitupa M, Louheranta A, Lindström J *et al*. The Finnish Diabetes Prevention Study. *Br J Nutr* 2000; **83 (Suppl 1)**: S137–42

63 Tuomilehto J, Lindström J, Eriksson J *et al*. Prevention of type 2 diabetes mellitus by changes in lifestyle among subjects with impaired glucose tolerance. *N Engl J Med* 2001; **344**: 1343–50

64 The Diabetes Prevention Program Research Group. The Diabetes Prevention Program. Design and methods for a clinical trial in the prevention of type 2 diabetes. *Diabetes Care* 1999; **22**: 623–34

65 National Institute of Diabetes and Digestive and Kidney Diseases. *Diet and Exercise Dramatically Delay Type 2 Diabetes*. Press release, August 8, 2001. http://www.niddk.nih.gov/welcome/releases/8_8_01.htm

66 Puska P, Tuomilehto J, Nissinen A, Vartiainen E. *The North Karelia Project. 20 Year Results and Experiences*. Helsinki: National Public Health Institute, 1995

Index